Handbook of
Movement
Disorders

Handbook of
Movement
Disorders

Stanley Fahn, MD

H. Houston Merritt Professor of
Neurology
College of Physicians & Surgeons
of Columbia University
New York City, New York

Paul E. Greene, MD

Assistant Professor
Department of Neurology
College of Physicians & Surgeons
of Columbia University
New York City, New York

Blair Ford, MD, FRCP(C)

Assistant Professor
Department of Neurology
College of Physicians & Surgeons
of Columbia University
New York City, New York

Susan B. Bressman, MD

Associate Professor
Department of Neurology
College of Physicians & Surgeons
of Columbia University
New York City, New York

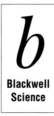

b

**Blackwell
Science**

Developed by **Current Medicine, Inc.**

Current Medicine, Inc.

400 Market Street, Suite 700
Philadelphia, PA 19106

Managing Editor	Lori Bainbridge
Development Editor	Gloria Klaiman
Art Director	Paul Fennessy
Cover Design, Interior Design and Layout	Lisa Adamitis
Illustration Director	Ann Saydlowski
Illustrators	Liz Carrozza, Ann Saydlowski, Beth Starkey, Lisa Weischedel, and Debra Wertz
Production	Lori Holland and Sally Nicholson
Indexing	Alexandra Nickerson

Library of Congress Cataloging-in-Publication Data
Handbook of movement disorders/Stanley Fahn...(et al.)
     p. cm.
     Includes bibliographical references and index
ISBN 1-57340-110-2
1. Movement disorders—Handbooks, manuals, etc. I. Fahn, Stanley, 1933-
(DNLM: 1. Movement Disorders—handbooks. WL 39 H2366 1997)
RC376.5.H35 1997
DNLM/DLC   97-31216
for Library of Congress   CIP

Every effort has been made to ensure that the drug dosage schedules within this text are accurate and conform to standards at the time of publication. However, as treatment recommendations vary in the light of continuing research and clinical experience, the reader is advised to verify drug dosage schedules herein with information found on product information sheets. This is especially true in cases of new or infrequently used drugs.

Printed in the United States by Quebecor Printing

10 9 8 7 6 5 4 3 2 1

PREFACE

Developments in the field of movement disorders are progressing at a rapid pace. It is now quite a challenge to educate neurologists and others in the medical profession about the current status of many of the disorders comprising movement disorders, and to keep the discourse brief and easy to comprehend.

We have undertaken this task by creating a *Handbook of Movement Disorders* that presents the most important material in a condensed fashion, with a maximum number of figures and tables, and a minimum amount of text—enough to keep the reader on targret as to the essential points. Rather than create many new figures, we have relied heavily upon the medical literature as a valuable resource, and we appreciate all the effort that the originators of these valuable sources had undertaken; we acknowledge the sources and thank the authors and publishers for allowing us to use them in this document.

We are not certain how long it will take readers to cover this *Handbook* from beginning to end, but we have endeavored to draw them into this volume by keeping both the text and the accompanying figures and tables lucid and memorable. Our goal is to educate readers and to provide them with an approach to the field of movement disorders that results in better care of their patients.

Stanley Fahn
Paul E. Greene
Blair Ford
Susan B. Bressman

CONTENTS

Chapter 9

Chapter 10

INTRODUCTION

◆ Epidemiology

◆ Evaluation of a Movement Disorder

Movement disorders can be defined as neurologic syndromes in which there is either an excess of movement (commonly referred to as *hyperkinesia, dyskinesia,* and *abnormal involuntary movement*) or a paucity of voluntary and automatic movements, unrelated to weakness or spasticity. The latter group can be referred to as *hypokinesia* (decreased amplitude of movement), but *bradykinesia* (slowness of movement) and *akinesia* (loss of movement) are common alternatives. The parkinsonian syndromes are the most common cause of such paucity of movement; other hypokinetic disorders represent only a small group of patients. Basically, movement disorders can be conveniently divided into parkinsonism and all other types. Gait can be affected by most types of movement disorders, including parkinsonism, dystonia, chorea, myoclonus, and cerebellar ataxia (Table 1-1).

Most movement disorders are associated with pathologic alterations in the basal ganglia or their connections. The basal ganglia are that group of gray matter nuclei lying deep within the cerebral hemispheres (caudate, putamen, and globus pallidus), the diencephalon (subthalamic nucleus), and the mesencephalon (substantia nigra). There are some exceptions to this general rule. Disease of the cerebellum or its pathways typically results in impairment of coordination (asynergy, ataxia), misjudgment of distance (dysmetria), and intention tremor. Myoclonus and many forms of tremors do not appear to be related primarily to basal ganglia pathology and often arise elsewhere in the central nervous system, including cerebral cortex (cortical reflex myoclonus), brain stem (reticular reflex myoclonus, hyperekplexia, and rhythmical brain stem myoclonus such as palatal myoclonus and ocular myoclonus), and spinal cord (rhythmical segmental myoclonus and nonrhythmic propriospinal myoclonus). Moreover, many myoclonic disorders are associated with diseases in which the cerebellum is involved, such as those causing the Ramsay Hunt syndrome. It is not known for certain which part of the brain is associated with tics, although the basal ganglia and the limbic structures have been implicated. Specific movement disorders are classically associated with certain loca-

Table 1-1. List of Movement Disorders

Hypokinesias

*Akinesia/bradykinesia (parkinsonism)

Catatonia, psychomotor depression,
  and obsessional slowness

Freezing phenomenon

Hypothyroid slowness

Stiff muscles

Hyperkinesias

Abdominal dyskinesias

Akathitic movements

Asynergia/ataxia

Athetosis

Ballism

*Chorea

Dysmetria

Hyperkinesias (*continued*)

*Dystonia

Hemifacial spasm

Hyperekplexia

Hypnogenic dyskinesias

Jumpy stumps

Moving toes/fingers

*Myoclonus

Myokymia

Myorhythmia

Paroxysmal dyskinesias

Restless legs

Stereotypy

*Tics

*Tremor

*Other than the cerebellar disorders (indicated by asynergia/ataxia and
dysmetria) these movement disorders are the most commonly encountered
in neurology.

tions within the basal ganglia: bradykinesia and rest tremor in the substantia nigra; ballism in the subthalamic nucleus; chorea in the caudate
nucleus; and dystonia in the putamen. Some Movement Disorders derive
from the peripheral nerve or its more proximal parts, the nerve roots or
motoneuron perikarya. Hemifacial spasm, myokymia, and the muscle
spasms (stiff muscles) of Isaacs syndrome are the most well recognized.
Others are the jumpy stumps and moving toes (fingers)/painful legs (arms)
syndromes. The former is seen in some amputees; the latter as a complication to some injury to peripheral nerves or roots (Fig. 1-1).

A large number of movement disorders are genetic in cause. Some of these
diseases have now been mapped to specific regions of the genome, and
some have even been localized to a specific gene (Fig. 1-2, Table 1-2).

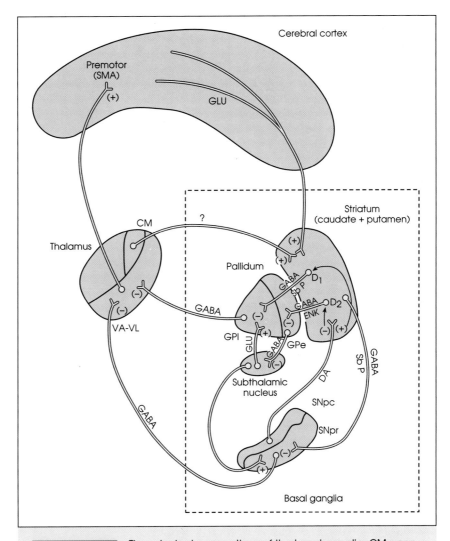

FIGURE 1-1 The principal connections of the basal ganglia. CM—centromedian nucleus of thalamus; D_1—dopamine receptor, type 1; D_2—dopamine receptor, type 2; DA—dopamine; ENK—enkephalin; GABA—γ aminobutyric acid; GLU—glutamate; GPe—globus pallidus external segment; GPI—globus pallidus internal segment; SbP—substance P; SMA—supplementary motor area; SNpc—substantia nigra, pars compacta; SNpr—substantia nigra, pars reticulata; VA-VL—ventroanterior and ventrolateral nuclei of thalamus; pallidum (=globus pallidus). (*Adapted from* Lang and colleague (1); with permission.)

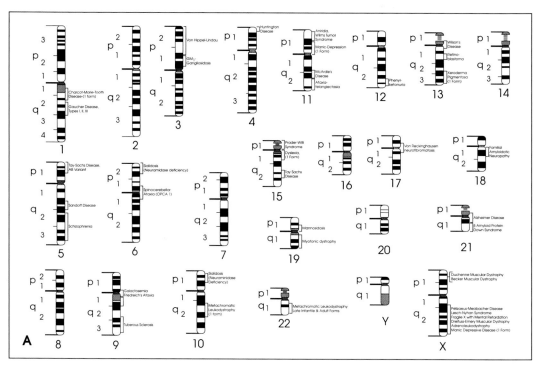

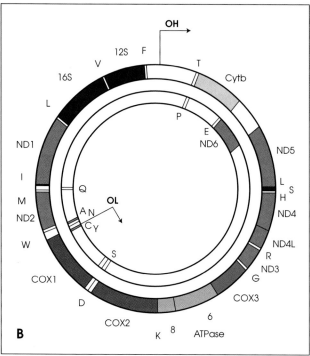

FIGURE 1-2 **A,** Gene map for movement disorders. **B,** Human mitochondrial DNA. (Panel A *adapted from* Martin (2); with permission; Panel B *adapted from* Tritschler and colleague (3); with permission.)

Table 1-2. Gene Map for Movement Disorders

Chromosome	Disease	Location	Inheritance mode
Chromosome 3	Hereditary spinocerebellar ataxia, type 7 (SCA7)	3p14–21.1	AD
Chromosome 4	Huntington's disease	4p16.3	AD
Chromosome 5	Hereditary hyperekplexia	5q	AD
Chromosome 6	Hereditary spinocerebellar ataxia, type 1 (SCA1)	6p23–p24	AD
	Juvenile myoclonic epilepsy	6p	AD
Chromosome 9	Idiopathic torsion dystonia	9q34	AD
	Friedreich's ataxia	9q13–q21.1	AR
Chromosome 11	Ataxia-telangiectasia	11q22–q23	AR
	Hereditary spinocerebellar ataxia, type 5 (SCA5)	11 centromere	AD
Chromosome 12	Dentatorubropallidoluysian atrophy (DRPLA)	12p12	AD
	Paroxysmal ataxia/myokymia	12p13	AD
	Hereditary spinocerebellar ataxia, type 2 (SCA2)	12q23–24	AD
Chromosome 13	Wilson's disease	13q14.3	AR
Chromosome 14	Dopa-responsive dystonia (DRD)	14q22.1–2	AD
	Hereditary spinocerebellar ataxia, type 3 (SCA3)	14q24–32	AD
	Machado-Joseph disease (types 1, 2, and 3)	14q32.1	AD
Chromosome 16	Herditary spinocerebellar ataxia, type 4 (SCA4)	16q24	AD
Chromosome 17	Disinhibition-dementia-parkinsonism-amyotrophy complex	17q21–23	AD
Chromosome 20	Familial Creutzfeldt-Jakob disease	20p terminal-p12	AD
Chromosome 21	Familial amyotrophic lateral sclerosis (ALS)	21q	AD
	Unverricht-Lundborg disease	21q22.3	AD
Chromosome X	Lubag (X-linked dystonia-parkinsonism)	Xq13	X-linked
	Lesch-Nyhan disease	Xq26–q27.2	X-linked
Mitochondrial DNA	Leigh disease	bp 8993 mutation (ATPase, subunit 6)	Usually sporadic
	Neuropathy, ataxia, retinitis pigmentosa (NARP)	bp 8993 mutation (ATPase, subunit 6)	Maternal
	Mitochondrial encephalopathy with ragged red fibers (MERRF)	tRNA^{lys} gene	Maternal

AD—autosomal dominant; AR—autosomal recessive.

Table 1-3. Prevalence of Movement Disorders

Essential tremor	415
Parkinson's disease	187
Tourette syndrome	29–1052
Dystonia	33
Hemifacial spasm	7.4–14.5
Hereditary ataxia	6
Huntington's disease	2–12
Multiple system atrophies	2
Wilson's disease	3
Progressive supranuclear palsy	2

Rates are given per 100,000 population. For Parkinson's disease, the rate is 347 per 100,000 for ages over 40 years. (From Schoenberg and colleagues [4]; with permission.)

Epidemiology

Movement disorders are fairly common neurologic problems but epidemiologic studies are lacking for many of them. Table 1-3 lists the prevalence rates of some of the movement disorders based on studies in the United States.

Evaluation of a Movement Disorder

The first question to be answered when seeing a patient for the possible presence of abnormal movements is whether or not involuntary movements are actually present. One must decide if the suspected abnormal movements might be purposeful voluntary movements, such as exaggerated gestures, mannerisms, or compulsive movements, or if the sustained contracted muscles might be "involuntary" muscle tightness to reduce pain (so-called "guarding"). As a general rule, abnormal involuntary movements are exaggerated with anxiety and diminished during sleep. They may or may not lessen with amobarbital or with hypnosis.

Table 1-4. Clinical Clues to Differentiate Some Common Movement Disorders

Rhythmical movements
  Tremor
      Resting
      Postural
      Action
      Intention
  Myoclonus, segmental
  Moving toes/fingers
  Dystonic tremor
  Periodic movements in sleep
  Tardive dyskinesia

Sustained movements
  Dystonia
  Stiff-person syndrome

Intermittent movements
  Paroxysmal dyskinesias (*eg*, kinesigenic induced)
  Tics

Speed of movements
  Myoclonus > chorea > athetosis

Suppressibility of movements
  Tics > chorea > dystonia > tremor

Complex movements
  Tics, stereotypies, psychogenic, and akathitic movements

Once it has been decided that abnormal involuntary movements are present and which body parts are involved, the next question is to determine the category of the involuntary movement, such as chorea, dystonia, myoclonus, tics, and tremor. In other words, one must determine the nature of the involuntary movements. To do so, one evaluates features such as rhythmicity, speed, duration, pattern (*eg*, repetitive, flowing, continual, paroxysmal, diurnal), induction (*ie*, stimuli-induced, action-induced, exercise-induced), complexity of the movements (complex vs simple), suppressibility by volitional attention or by sensory tricks, and whether the movements are accompanied by sensations such as restlessness or the urge to make a movement that can release a built-up tension (Table 1-4).

References

1. Lang AE, Weiner W: *Movement Disorders: A Comprehensive Survey*. Mount Kisco, NY: Futura; 1989; 1–22.
2. Martin JB: Molecular genetic studies in the neuropsychiatric disorders. *Trends in Neurosciences* 1989, 12:130–137.
3. Tritschler H-J, Medori R: Mitochondrial DNA alterations as a source of human disorders. *Neurology* 1993, 43:280–288.
4. Schoenberg BS, Anderson DW, Haerer AF: Prevalence of Parkinson's disease in the population of Copiah County, Mississippi. *Neurology* 1985, 35:841–845.

Chapter 2

PARKINSONISM

◆ Definition

◆ Classification

◆ Parkinson's Disease

◆ Parkinson Plus Syndromes

Definition

The term *parkinsonism* is applied to neurologic syndromes in which patients exhibit some combination of rest tremor, rigidity, bradykinesia, and loss of postural reflexes. Patients with all these clinical features are likely to have a disturbance of the nigrostriatal dopamine system. In patients who lack one or two of these major features, the presence of dopaminergic dysfunction is less certain. Many patients with parkinsonism may also have other characteristic signs and symptoms. For example, in the "freezing" phenomenon, patients experience a sudden transient inability to move one or both feet. This may happen on gait initiation, during turning, at boundaries (curbs, doorways, and so on), on reaching a destination, and when startled or under emotional pressure. When severe, freezing episodes can lead to frequent falls and are a major source of disability. In some patients, freezing in the lower extremities is accompanied by a similar phenomenon during speaking, and in the upper extremities during writing or other fine motor movements (Table 2-1 and Fig. 2-1).

Classification

Parkinson's disease (PD) is the most common form of parkinsonism, occurring in about 200 per 100,000 people in the general population. However, a minority of patients with parkinsonism have a disturbance in the nigrostriatal system from another cause. Virtually every category of human disease can occasionally produce parkinsonism, including intoxications, tumors, infections, metabolic derangements, trauma, vascular disease, and degenerative diseases other than PD. Although many of these conditions produce signs and symptoms that do not occur in PD, up to 25% of patients with clinically diagnosed PD have been found to have another disease at autopsy [1] (Table 2-2).

Table 2-1. Characteristics of Parkinsonism

Major features

Rest tremor

Rigidity

Bradykinesia

Loss of postural reflexes

Flexed posture

Variable features

Motor	Autonomic	Cognitive	Other
Freezing of gait	Urinary frequency	Slowness in thinking	Glabellar, palmomental, snout reflexes (frontal release signs)
Dystonia	Constipation	Dementia	Limitation of upgaze
Muscle ache	Impotence in men	Depression	Interruption of smooth ocular pursuit
Kyphosis			Seborrhea

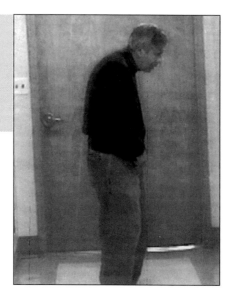

FIGURE 2-1 This patient with Parkinson's disease demonstrates the mild typical flexed (stooped) posture of this disease. Also note that the arms are held close to the body, and they are slightly flexed at the elbow.

Table 2-2. Classification of Parkinsonian Syndromes

Idiopathic (Lewy body) parkinsonism
Parkinson's disease

Secondary parkinsonism
Drug-induced
  Dopamine receptor blockers (neuroleptics, antiemetics)
  Dopamine depleters (reserpine, tetrabenazine)
  Lithium
  Flunarizine, cinnarizine, diltiazem
Hemiatrophy-Hemiparkinsonism
Hydrocephalus
  Normal pressure hypocephalus
  Noncommunicating hydrocephalus
Hypoxia
Infectious
  Fungal infection
  AIDS
  Subacute sclerosing panencephalitis
  Postencephalitic (encephalitis lethargica, other encephalitides)
  Creutzfeldt-Jakob disease
  Gerstmann-Strausler-Scheinker disease
Metabolic
  Hypocalcemic parkinsonism (basal ganglia calcification)
  Chronic hepatocerebral degeneration
  Wilson's disease
  Ceroid lipofuscinosis
  GM_1 gangliosidosis
  Gaucher's disease
  Mitochondrial encephalomyopathies
Paraneoplastic parkinsonism
Psychogenic parkinsonism
Syringomesencephalia
Trauma (boxers encephalopathy)

(*Continued on next page*)

Table 2-2. (*continued*)

Toxin
  MPTP (1-methyl-4-phenyl-1,2,3,6-tetrahydropyridine) intoxication
    Carbon monoxide intoxication
  Manganese intoxication
  Cyanide intoxication
  Methanol intoxication
  Carbon disulfide intoxication
  Disulfiram intoxication
Tumor
  Vascular
  Multi-infarct
  Binswanger's disease

Parkinson-plus syndromes

Multiple System Atrophy Syndromes (MSA)
  Striatonigral degeneration
  Shy-Drager syndrome
  Sporadic olivopontocerebellar atrophy
Steele-Richardson-Olszewski disease (SRO or PSP)
Cortical basal ganglionic degeneration
Progressive pallidal atrophy
Lytico-Bodig (Guamanian PD-D-ALS)
Motor neuron disease-Parkinsonism
Dementia syndromes
  Alzheimer's Disease
  Cortical (Diffuse) Lewy body disease
  Pick's Disease

Heredodegenerative diseases

Hallervorden-Spatz disease
Huntington's disease
Lubag (Filipino X-linked dystonia-parkinson)
Machado-Joseph Azorean disease
Neuroacanthocytosis
Familial olivopontocerebellar
Thalamic dementia syndrome
Neuronal intranuclear hyaline inclusion diseases

Parkinson's Disease

Usually, the diagnosis of PD is suggested by history, clinical examination, and the absence of incompatible clinical, laboratory, or radiologic abnormalities. However, no single feature absolutely guarantees or excludes the diagnosis of PD. A dramatic response to levodopa is virtually universal in patients with PD, but occasionally occurs early in the course of other Parkinson syndromes such as olivopontocerebellar atrophy or progressive supranuclear palsy. Conversely, some patients with PD develop severe nausea, orthostatic hypotension, or psychosis at moderate doses of levodopa and are mistakenly diagnosed as having another Parkinson syndrome on the basis of levodopa failure. At the onset of the disease, patients with PD usually have symptoms limited to one side of the body (hemi-PD), although symptoms eventually spread to both sides of the body. Occasionally PD begins with symmetric symptoms. In addition, mass lesions such as tumors may compress the substantia nigra or putamen and produce unilateral parkinsonism (Table 2-3).

Motor Symptoms

The broad categories of tremor, rigidity, and bradykinesia do not do justice to the complex motor difficulties of patients with PD. Tremor can affect most voluntary muscles, including muscles of the face, tongue, jaw, upper and lower extremities and less commonly trunk and neck. The tremor is occasionally felt before it can be seen ("inner motor"), is present at rest, but can also be present with action. The tremor is sometimes

---

Table 2-3. Clinical Manifestations of Parkinson's Disease

Unilateral onset (hemiparkinsonism)

Rest tremor

Absence of other neurologic signs, such as spasticity, Babinski signs, atypical speech disturbance, etc.

Absence of laboratory or radiologic abnormalities

Slow progression

Dramatic response to levodopa

Preservation of postural reflexes early in the illness

severe enough to cause diaphoresis and weight loss. Rigidity contributes to slowness of movement, but patients with PD may be slow even when rigidity is minimal. Rigid muscles may be painful, and shoulder, calf, or thigh pain is sometimes the first symptom of PD. Bradykinesia manifests in multiple ways: decreased blinking and loss of facial expression (masked facies), decreased automatic swallowing leading to drooling, loss of arm swing while walking, and soft voice (hypophonia). During walking, some patients take faster and faster steps as the step size becomes smaller (festination) (Table 2-4). A similar phenomenon may affect writing or other repetitive movements (tachykinesia) (Figs. 2-2–2-6).

Table 2-4. Motor Symptoms of Parkinson's Disease

Tremor
  "Inner motor"
  Rest tremor
  Rest tremor persisting with action
  Action tremor (in addition to rest tremor)
Rigidity

Akinesia/Bradykinesia
  Decreased blink rate
  Facial masking
  Hypophonia
  Drooling
  Tachykinesia
  Terminal micrographia
  Festination
Loss of postural reflexes
Other motor features
  Dystonia
  Early morning dystonia, usually in the toes
  Hemidystonia
  Freezing
  Start hesitation
  Freezing of gait: during turning, at boundaries, at target, in mid-stride
  Freezing of other activities: speech (palilalia), writing

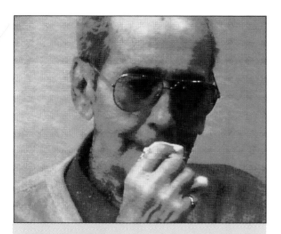

FIGURE 2-2 Drooling of saliva in a patient with a moderate degree of Parkinson's disease. Such patients tend to carry a handkerchief with them at all times.

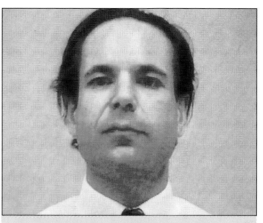

FIGURE 2-3 Flattening of the left nasolabial fold in a patient with predominantly left hemiparkinsonism.

FIGURE 2-4 Anterior displacement of the head (antecollis) in a patient with long-standing Parkinson's disease.

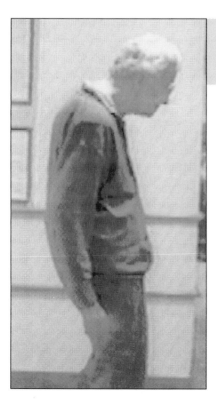

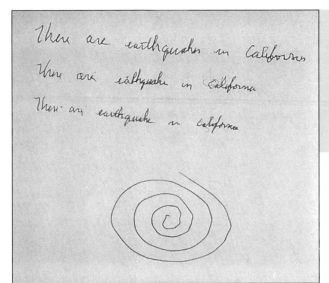

FIGURE 2-5 Handwriting sample of a patient with mild Parkinson's disease. Handwriting is slower and smaller (micrographia) in Parkinson's disease. The Archimedes spiral tends to be cramped and less open. Tremor, if present, can usually be seen in the writing.

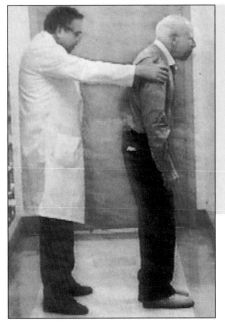

FIGURE 2-6 Demonstrating the pull test. The examiner stands behind the patient and pulls the patient backwards. After explaining that the patient should take a step backwards to prevent falling, the examiner gives a quick pull on the shoulders and tests for retropulsion. On the first attempt, it is advisable to use only mild to moderate force when pulling. If the patient recovers well, then a stronger pull is used. The patient may require a practice with a mild pull to appreciate what is expected of him. The examiner needs to be prepared to catch the patient should he not recover his balance. If the patient is larger than the examiner, it is wise to have a wall behind the examiner to keep both the patient and examiner from falling.

Pathology

The major pathologic abnormalities in PD are neuronal cell loss, gliosis, and loss of iron pigment in the substantia nigra, especially in the ventrolateral portion projecting to the putamen, and the presence of abnormal intracytoplasmic neuronal inclusions, called Lewy bodies. Lewy bodies consist of an amorphous central core with a halo of radially arranged 10- to 20-nm in diameter neurofilaments. Lewy bodies stain with monoclonal antibodies to ubiquitin (a polypeptide associated with protein degradation) and to selected antigens from tubulin, paired helical filaments, and neurofibrillary tangle proteins. In many patients with PD, ubiquitin staining has revealed the presence of cortical intracytoplasmic inclusions, which resemble Lewy bodies but are homogeneous in structure. Dopaminergic nuclei in the ventral tegmental area also show cell loss and Lewy body formation. Other neurotransmitter systems may undergo neuronal loss with Lewy bodies in PD, including noradrenergic neurons (locus ceruleus, dorsal nucleus of the vagus), cholinergic neurons (nucleus basalis of Meynert, Westphal-Edinger nucleus), and serotonergic neurons (dorsal raphe nucleus). Although damage in these systems is usually less severe than damage to the substantia nigra, some symptoms of PD that respond poorly to dopamine replacement therapy may result from damage to nondopaminergic systems (Fig. 2-7).

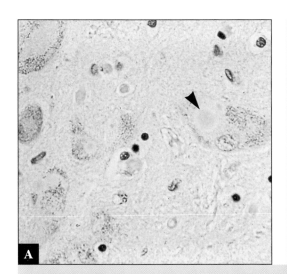
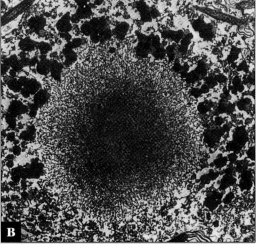

FIGURE 2-7 **A,** Lewy bodies in the substantia nigra (*arrow*) (*See* Color Plate). Hematoxylin and eosin stain. **B,** Electron microscopy of Lewy body. The ultrastructure of the Lewy body consists of a homogeneous core surrounded by radiating filaments (magnification x 2000).

Neuroimaging

Computed tomography (CT) and magnetic resonance imaging (MRI) are useful for identifying some causes of parkinsonism, but they generally yield normal results in PD. It is difficult to detect MRI abnormalities in the substantia nigra corresponding to the cell loss or iron deposition that occur in PD, although there have been occasional reports of abnormalities in other forms of parkinsonism. MRI at a higher magnetic field strength may allow more sensitive detection of iron and gliosis and may eventually play a larger role in clinical evaluation of PD. Positron emission tomography (PET) imaging using fluorodopa is sensitive to loss of dopamine, and demonstrates a marked decrease in striatal fluorodopa uptake in patients with PD (Fig. 2-8).

Physiology of the Basal Ganglia

Idiopathic PD develops when neurons in the substantia nigra pars compacta degenerate and levels of dopamine decrease in the putamen and caudate nuclei. The loss of dopamine upsets the balance between excitatory and inhibitory pathways in the basal ganglia. Although dopamine stimulates both excitatory and inhibitory output within the putamen, the ultimate effect of reduced dopamine is increased output from the internal segment of the globus pallidus. This output is itself inhibitory, and turns

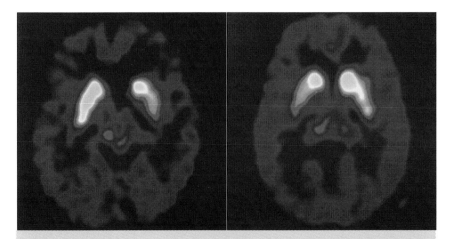

FIGURE 2-8 Fluorodopa positron emission tomography (PET) scans in a patient with predominantly right-sided Parkinson's disease (*left*) and in a patient with more bilateral involvement (*right*). The posterior putamen in PD shows more reduced levodopa uptake than other parts of the striatum. Asymmetry can be seen even in the right PET scan, with more pronounced reduction in the right putamen. (*See* Color Plate.)

off the ventrolateral thalamus, which is the major target of the motor output pathway of the basal ganglia. The effects of decreased dopamine are mediated by increased output from the subthalamic nucleus and the internal segment of the globus pallidus; this process has stimulated attempts to undo the effects of dopamine deficiency by surgical lesions in those structures (Fig. 2-9).

Etiology and Pathogenesis

The cause for degeneration of the substantia nigra in PD remains unknown. Some explanations currently considered include intoxication by an endogenous or environmental toxicant, or a genetic predisposition. None of the current proposals explains all the features of PD as we know it, although each explains some aspects of the disease, and each hypothesis is actively being investigated by its proponents. The toxicant MPTP (1-methyl-4-phenyl-1,2,3,6-tetrahydropyridine) produces a condition in people and animals that resembles PD both clinically and pathologically. No similar toxin in the environment has yet been identified. Oxidation of dopamine in the substantia nigra is known to produce oxygen radicals that are toxic to cells. There is indirect evidence that patients with PD may not be able to detoxify these radicals adequately, which might produce the ongoing neuronal damage that occurs in PD. Attempts to retard the progression of PD using antioxidants have not yet proven beneficial. A twin study done in 1981 [2] indicated a low concordance of PD in monozygotic twins, which initially discouraged attempts to find a genetic basis for PD. Case-controlled studies, however, have shown that relatives of patients with PD have a higher risk of developing the disease than nonrelatives. Reanalysis of the original twin data, including abnormal PET scans of apparently "asymptomatic" twins and subsequent development of PD in some originally asymptomatic twins, has renewed the search for a genetic component to PD. As might be expected, it has also been suggested that a combination of factors, such as an inherited predisposition to an environmental toxicant, may actually explain PD (Figs. 2-10 and 2-11). In a large Italian and several smaller Greek families with autosomal dominant Parkinson's disease, a mutation in the gene for the synaptic protein, α-synuclein, on chromosome 4q has been discovered.

Treatment of Uncomplicated Parkinson's Disease

Levodopa is the single most effective symptomatic treatment for patients with PD. It is usually administered as carbidopa/levodopa, a combination of levodopa and the peripheral-acting dopamine decarboxylase inhibitor carbidopa, which increases penetration of levodopa into the

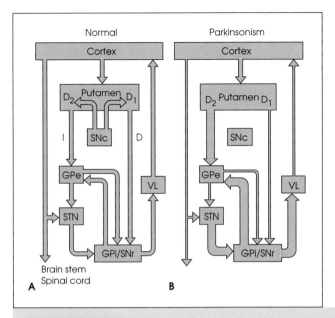

FIGURE 2-9 Pathophysiology of the basal ganglia in Parkinson's disease. **A,** Dopamine from the substantia nigra pars compacta (SNc) innervates the neostriatum, with a mechanism affecting the "indirect" and "direct" pathways. Dopamine inhibits the striatal neurons via D_2 receptors belonging to the indirect pathway. These striatal GABA-ergic neurons send inhibitory output fibers to the globus pallidus externa (GPe); the GPe sends GABA-ergic inhibitory fibers to the subthalamic nucleus (STN); the STN sends glutamatergic excitatory fibers to the globus pallidus interna (GPi); the GPi sends GABA-ergic inhibitory fibers to the ventrolateral (VL) and ventral anterior (VA) nuclei of the thalamus. The net effect of dopamine via the indirect pathway is to inhibit the tonically active GPi. Conversely, dopamine excites, via D_1 receptors, the striatal neurons belonging to the direct pathway. These striatal GABA-ergic neurons send inhibitory output fibers directly to the GPi. The net effect of dopamine via the direct pathway is to inhibit the tonically active GPi. Thus, by both the indirect and direct pathways, the GPi is inhibited by dopamine acting through the striatum. **B,** In Parkinson's disease, with loss of striatal dopamine due to degeneration of the substantia nigra pars compacta neurons, the net effect is to increase the activity of the GPi by both the indirect and direct pathways. Open arrows—excitatory connections; filled arrows—inhibitory connections. (*Adapted from* Wichmann and colleague (3).)

brain and decreases dopamine-induced side effects outside the brain. Nonetheless, patients taking high doses of levodopa often develop complications of therapy (see the next section). It has been suggested that levodopa itself promotes development of such complications. Although this has never been established, it seems prudent to use alternative medications when possible, minimizing the dose of levodopa when it is needed. Patients with mild PD may not need any medications, although they may benefit from treatment of related conditions such as depres-

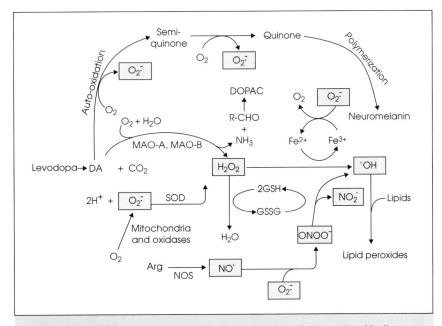

FIGURE 2-10 Dopamine metabolism pathways that can lead to the synthesis of hydrogen peroxide and the oxyradicals, superoxide and hydroxyl radical, and showing the possible contribution of nitric oxide in reacting with superoxide radical to form other free radicals. The free radicals and H_2O_2 are highlighted within rectangles. Arg—arginine; DA—dopamine; DOPAC—dihydroxyphenylacetic acid; GSH—reduced glutathione; GSSG—oxidized glutathione; H_2O_2—hydrogen peroxide; MAO—monoamine oxidase; NH_3—ammonia; NOS—nitric oxide synthase; NO—nitric oxide radical; OH—hydroxyl radical; O_2^-—superoxide anion radical; ONOO—peroxynitrite; R-CHO—dopa aldehyde; SOD—superoxide dismutase.

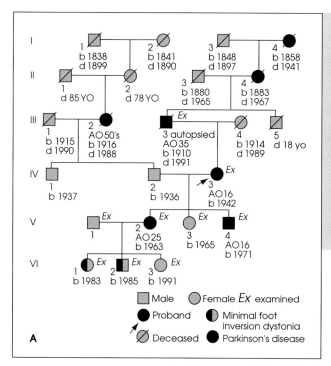

FIGURE 2-11 Pedigrees of families with autosomal dominant Parkinson's disease. **A,** A pedigree of a family with autosomal dominant Parkinson's disease. This family has been shown to have a mutation in the gene on chromosome 4q for the synaptic protein, α-synuclein. **B,** Pedigrees of three families with Parkinson's disease compatible with autosomal dominant transmission with reduced penetrance. (Panel A *adapted from* Golbe and colleagues (4); panel B *adapted from* Lazzarini and colleagues (5).)

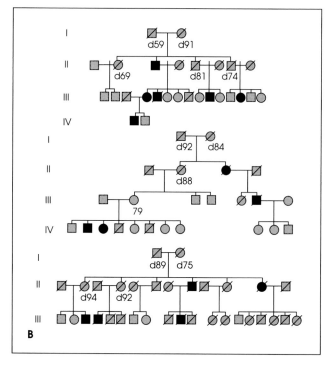

sion. In such patients, it would be ideal to prevent progression of the disease. The monoamine oxidase (MAO)-B inhibitor selegiline was found to delay the need for levodopa in patients with mild PD, but this effect was probably due to its prolonged symptomatic effect rather than a true protective effect. For patients requiring symptomatic relief, but whose symptoms are still mild, a variety of other medications are available. Amantadine promotes release of dopamine from remaining nigral neurons and provides relief of symptoms in about two thirds of patients. Anticholinergic medications cause memory loss and confusion in older individuals, but often reduce tremor when tolerated. Dopamine agonists provide modest but long-lasting symptomatic relief, especially when added to levodopa.

Motor Complications of Parkinson's Disease

Patients treated with levodopa initially generally experience long-lasting improvement in motor symptoms after each dose of levodopa. With time, many patients develop progressive reduction in the duration of benefit from each dose of medication ("wearing off"). As patients develop wearing off, many also develop troublesome involuntary movements (dyskinesia or dystonia) in response to each dose of levodopa. These involuntary movements usually occur as the blood level of levodopa peaks ("peak dose" dyskinesias), or less commonly, at the beginning and end of the dosing period (called *dyskinesia-improvement-dyskinesia* [DID]). As the dyskinesia or dystonia worsens, the threshold for the appearance of levodopa-induced movements approaches the dose required to produce a benefit, leaving an extremely narrow window between Parkinson symptoms and excess movement. In addition, some patients develop a variety of other fluctuations, including sudden loss of benefit ("on/off"), sudden change from severe dyskinesias to severe Parkinson symptoms ("yo/yo"), loss of benefit after a protein meal, and failure of an occasional dose of levodopa to produce benefit ("dose failure") (Fig. 2-12).

Treatment of Complicated Parkinson's Disease

When dyskinesias become severe, the amount of levodopa taken at each dose must be decreased. To titrate the dose more accurately, levodopa can be given without carbidopa, or carbidopa/levodopa can be dissolved in water acidified with vitamin C. Sometimes, each individual dose of levodopa becomes so small that no benefit results. Some patients may do better using longer acting agents such as time-release carbidopa/levodopa or dopamine agonists. Patients with intolerable offs may achieve a rapid response from the injectable medication apomorphine, or by crushing the pill and taking it with liquid to speed up entry into the small intestine. Because levodopa is not absorbed from the stomach, delay in gastric emptying may produce an apparent failure to respond to a dose of levodopa in a patient who otherwise does well; this also may improve when the pill is dissolved in liquid. When patients do develop severe dyskinesias or dystonia, adding dopamine agonists and reducing the dose of levodopa often provides a smoother response and less severe involuntary movements than levodopa alone. When this fails, the atypical neuroleptic clozapine sometimes reduces dyskinesias without worsening PD symptoms. Surgical pallidotomy also may reduce levodopa-induced involuntary movements (see the next section). Freezing is usually relieved by increased medication. However, freezing occasionally persists in someone who is otherwise adequately treated, and sometimes even worsens as medication is increased. Rarely, anti-Parkinson medications such as amantadine and levodopa may produce myoclonus that is severe enough to interfere with function. Patients with PD may have myoclonus even in the absence of medication, but these patients often have dementia as well, and the diagnosis of PD may be incorrect (Figs. 2-13 and 2-14, Table 2-5).

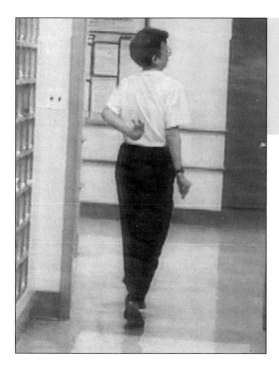

FIGURE 2-12 A patient with Parkinson's disease having peak dose choreic and dystonic movements. The left arm excessively swings and goes behind her back as the patient is walking. The dyskinesias are more pronounced on the side of the body that has the more severe parkinsonism.

Neurosurgical Treatment of Parkinson's Disease

Several neurosurgical procedures are currently being used to treat PD. Surgical lesions in the output pathways from the basal ganglia have been used to treat PD since the 1950s. Stereotactically placed lesions in the ventrolateral thalamus (thalamotomy) may produce dramatic relief of tremor, but are less effective in reducing rigidity and bradykinesia. Bilateral thalamic lesions may produce speech and swallowing disturbances. Lesions in the posteroventral globus pallidus (pallidotomy) dramatically reduce levodopa-induced dyskinesias, and may be more effective than thalamotomy in reducing bradykinesia. In a different surgical approach, dopamine-producing tissue such as fetal mesencephalic tissue can be surgically implanted into dopamine target areas in the putamen and caudate nuclei. In addition to providing a replacement for missing dopamine, transplanted tissue does establish functional connections with the host brain and may actually affect the course of the underlying disease. The long-term effects of pallidotomy and fetal tissue transplants are unknown (Figs. 2-15–2-17).

Parkinson Plus Syndromes

Progressive Supranuclear Palsy

Clinical Characteristics

The defining description of progressive supranuclear palsy (PSP) appeared in 1964 in an article by Steele and colleagues [6]. The prevalence of PSP has been estimated at 1.39 per 100,000. The mean age at onset is about 65 years, with a male preponderance in most series. Symptoms are

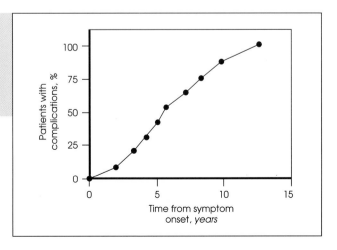

FIGURE 2-13 Time course for developing motor response complications in Parkinson's disease patients treated with levodopa. (*Adapted from* Chase and colleagues (7); with permission.)

steadily progressive; death, due to aspiration or the sequella of multiple falls or bed sores, usually occurs 5 to 10 years after onset. When supranuclear palsy (especially loss of downgaze) appears early in the course of an akinetic-rigid syndrome, the diagnosis of PSP is likely. PSP may be suspected in the absence of a supranuclear palsy when other typical features are present. Frequent or continuous square-wave jerks (small saccades alternately to the left and right in the horizontal plane) are often present. Patients with PSP lose postural reflexes early in the course, and falling is an early feature. While walking, patients often assume a broad base, abduct the upper extremities at the shoulder, and flex at the elbows, producing a gait that is characteristic of PSP. Freezing (abrupt, transient interruption of motor activity) may be severe, and in some cases may be the major manifestation of PSP. Facial dystonia (deep nasolabial folds and furrowed brow) may create an angry or puzzled look when combined with a wide-eyed, unblinking stare. Axial rigidity is often more prominent than rigidity of the extremities, and, in some cases, the limbs may have normal or reduced tone. Patients may be unable to open their eyelids even in

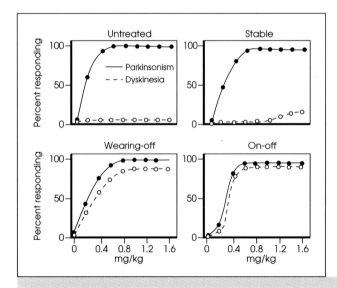

FIGURE 2-14 Levodopa dose-response curves in patients with Parkinson's disease who have never been treated, who have a stable response, who have "wearing-off," and who have "on-off." Curves with *solid circles* represent the parkinsonian motor responsiveness; curves with *open circles* represent the development of dyskinesias. In patients without fluctuations, benefit appears before dyskinesias. Once patients develop wearing-off and on-off, most patients develop dyskinesias at the doses required to produce benefit. These patients have a narrow therapeutic window. (*Adapted from* Mouradian and colleagues (8); with permission.)

Table 2-5. Treatment of Motor Complications of Levodopa Therapy

Problems with response fluctuations	Possible solution
Wearing off	Controlled-release levodopa
	Dopamine agonist (bromocriptine, pergolide, pramipexole, ropinerole)
	Other long-acting agent (selegiline, amantadine, anticholinergic)
	More frequent doses, in smaller amounts to prevent dyskinesias
On/off	Treat as if wearing off, use liquid levodopa or apomorphine for rapid on
Yo-yo	Use dopamine agonist as main agent with tiny amounts of levodopa/carbidopa or even plain levodopa as "booster"
Dose failure	Crush levodopa/carbidopa and dissolve in large amount of liquid to promote transit through the stomach
Failure to respond after protein meal	Rearrange diet so that most protein is ingested at the end of the day—consult nutritionist to ensure balanced nutritional intake

Dyskinesias

Peak dose dyskinesias	Reduce the dose of carbidopa/levodopa and replace with other medications
Diphasic dyskinesias	Treat as for "yo-yo" above
Painful "off" dyskinesia/dystonia	Clozapine
	Amantadine
	Pallidotomy

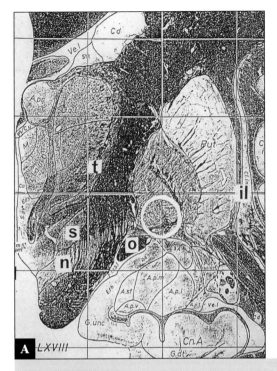
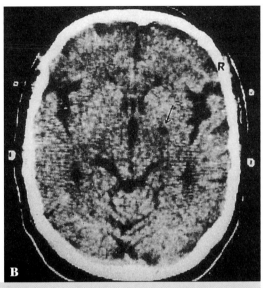

FIGURE 2-15 Pallidotomy in the posteroventral globus pallidus interna. **A**, Target for pallidotomy in the posteroventral globus pallidus interna. **B**, Computed tomography scan taken 6 months after a pallidotomy showing the location of the lesion. (*From* Laitinen and colleagues (9); with permission.)

the absence of orbicularis oculi spasms. This has been termed "apraxia of eyelid opening," but the phenomenon does not represent true apraxia, and it has been suggested that it is the result of inappropriate inhibition of the levator palpebrae [10] (Fig. 2-18–2-21).

Pathology

The pathology of PSP is characterized by cell loss and gliosis in the globus pallidus, subthalamic nucleus, red nucleus, substantia nigra, dentate nucleus, and the periaqueductal gray and tectum of the brain stem. Neurofibrillary tangles consisting of 15-nm straight filaments distinct from the tangles of Alzheimer's disease are found in the same areas, but may also be found diffusely in the brain stem. Senile plaques are not found. Recently, abnormal glia, with paired nuclei and fibrous inclusions, were found in PSP but not PD, striatonigral degeneration, or Alzheimer's disease. These inclusions, which stain with antibodies against the micro-

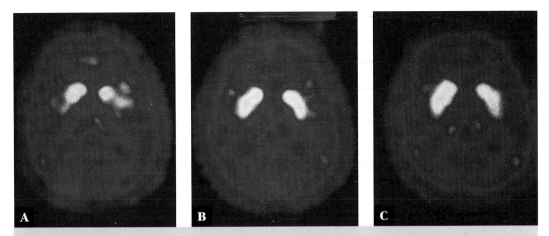

FIGURE 2-16 Fluorodopa PET scan before and after fetal mesencephalic tissue implant into the putamen of a patient with advanced Parkinson's disease (**A–C**). There is increased fluorodopa uptake 6 (*B*) and 12 (*C*) months after the transplant, whereas there was little uptake in the putamen prior to surgery (*A*). (*From* Kordower and colleagues (11); with permission.) (*See* Color Plate.)

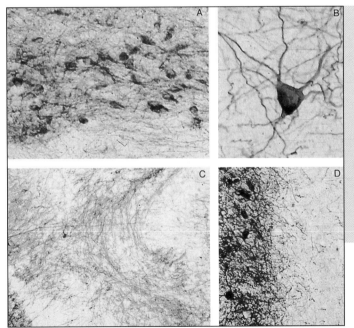

FIGURE 2-17 Post-mortem putamen stained for tyrosine hydroxylase of a patient with advanced Parkinson's disease who had a favorable response following fetal mesencephalic tissue implantation. The grafted neurons stain for the enzyme, indicating the production of dopamine. The grafted neurons have neuronal processes that are growing into the host's putamen. (*From* Kordower and colleagues (11); with permission.) (*See* Color Plate.)

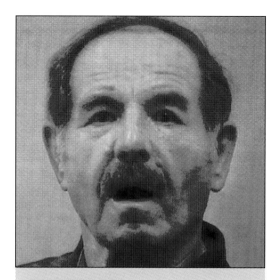

FIGURE 2-18 A patient with progressive supranuclear palsy, depicting the staring expression with eyes that barely move, deep nasolabial folds, and furrowed forehead and eyebrows, representing the "quizzical look."

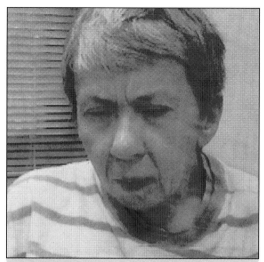

FIGURE 2-19 A patient with more advanced progressive supranuclear palsy. In addition to not being able to voluntarily move her eyes, the patient has blepharospasm (eyelid closure), furrowed brow, deep nasolabial folds, and a flexed head.

tubule-associated protein Tau, appear to differ from the glial inclusions described later in multiple system atrophy (Figs. 2-22 and 2-23).

Neuroimaging

Brain stem atrophy may be present on CT or MRI of patients with PSP, but this finding is neither sensitive nor specific. Decreased signal in the putamen detected with high-field strength, T2-weighted MRI may distinguish patients with PSP from normal subjects, but is more characteristic of multiple system atrophy syndromes. PET scanning currently provides the most useful neuroimaging tool. Imaging of dopamine uptake with ^{18}F-fluorodopa reveals a decrease in fluorodopa uptake in both the anterior and posterior putamen compared with uptake in PD, which is reduced in the posterior putamen, but less reduced in the anterior putamen and caudate nuclei. The overall severity of symptoms in PSP does not correlate with the reduction in fluorodopa uptake, highlighting the importance of pathologic changes outside the substantia nigra. PET scanning with ^{18}F-deoxyglucose reveals an anterior-to-posterior gradient, with greatest hypometabolism in the frontal cortex, and lesser degrees of hypometabolism in the striatum, thalamus, and cerebellum. Scanning with markers of dopamine D_2 binding in the striatum such as raclopride demonstrate a moderate reduction in dopamine-binding sites, but may be normal in some patients with PSP (Fig. 2-24).

Multiple System Atrophy

Clinical Characteristics

The term "multiple system atrophy" (MSA) was coined in 1969 by Graham and Oppenheimer in response to the observation that patients with

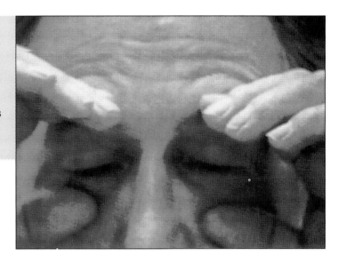

FIGURE 2-20 A patient with "apraxia" of eyelid opening due to progressive supranuclear palsy. He is attempting to open his eyelids after forcefully closing them on command. The inability to promptly open the eyelids leads the patient to use his fingers to pry them open.

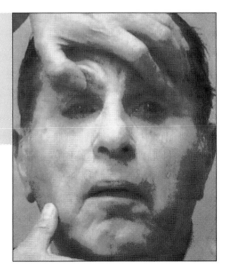

FIGURE 2-21 Testing of the oculocephalic reflexes (doll's eyes) to determine if the gaze palsy is supranuclear in origin. The patient is unable to look down voluntarily and is being asked to look straight ahead at an object while the examiner is tilting his head backward while keeping the eyelids apart to observe for the downward movement of the eyes. If the eyes move downward, the gaze palsy is supranuclear in etiology.

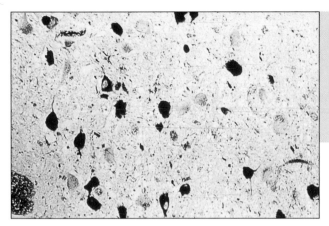

FIGURE 2-22 Neurofibrillary tangles in the locus ceruleus in a patient with progressive supranuclear palsy. This is a low power (magnification x 160) micrograph using a Gallyas (silver impregnation) technique. (*From* Lantos (12); with permission.)

a levodopa-unresponsive, akinetic-rigid syndrome plus cerebellar deficits or autonomic failure sometimes had widespread pathologic findings that could not be predicted on the basis of the clinical signs and symptoms [13]. These patients can be classified on clinical grounds as having Shy-Drager syndrome (SDS) if they have parkinsonism plus autonomic failure; olivopontocerebellar atrophy (OPCA) if they have parkinsonism plus cerebellar deficits; and striatonigral degeneration (SND) if they have levodopa-unresponsive parkinsonism without cerebellar signs, prominent autonomic dysfunction, or other abnormal neurologic findings. Although some patients classified as SDS, OPCA, or SND will eventually develop signs associated with the other syndromes, these categories are still useful as clinical labels, and the terms persist in general clinical use (Table 2-6, Fig. 2-25).

Pathology

The areas of pathologic involvement in MSA include Onuf's nucleus, pyramidal tracts, anterior horn cells, intermediolateral cell columns of the spinal cord, pontine nuclei, substantia nigra, locus ceruleus, inferior olives, dorsal motor nucleus of the vagus, vestibular nuclei, caudate, putamen, globus pallidus, and Purkinje cells. There is neuronal loss and gliosis in the involved areas, but neurofibrillary tangles and Lewy bodies are absent. Several reports have described cytoplasmic inclusions in glia and pontine neurons in the various MSA subtypes, which may not be found in other degenerative diseases (Fig. 2-26).

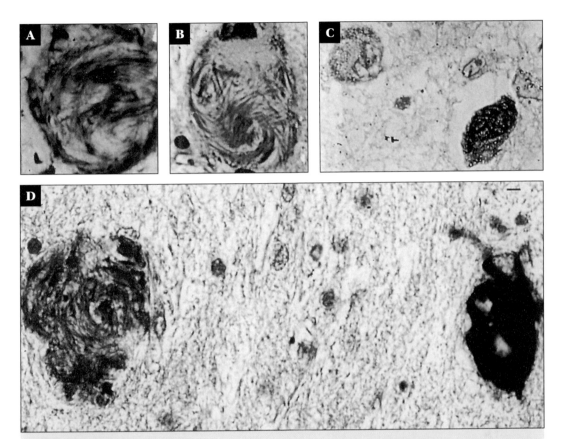

Neuroimaging

Computed tomography scanning in MSA may reveal focal atrophy of the cerebellum and brachium pontis, and the pattern of atrophy may be useful in subdividing types of OPCA. In addition, MRI may detect demyelination of the transverse pontine fibers. One study reported decreased glucose metabolism of the brain stem and cerebellum on PET scanning. SND can be difficult to distinguish from PD early in the course, due to the absence of marked cerebellar or autonomic deficits. Severe pathologic

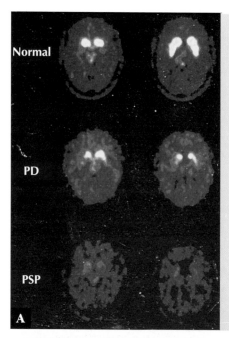

FIGURE 2-24 Fluorodopa and raclopride positron emission tomography (PET) scanning in progressive supranuclear palsy. A patient with progressive supranuclear palsy (PSP) and a patient with Parkinson's disease (PD) are compared with a normal control. **A**, There is a severe reduction of fluorodopa uptake in PSP, whereas in PD there is some uptake in the caudate nucleus. **B**, Raclopride is a dopamine D_2 receptor antagonist that is used to measure the number of available D_2 receptors. Raclopride PET scanning reveals a loss of D_2 receptors in the caudate and putamen in a patient with PSP, with normal numbers of D_2 receptors in a patient with PD. (*From* Brooks (15); with permission.) (*See* Color Plate.)

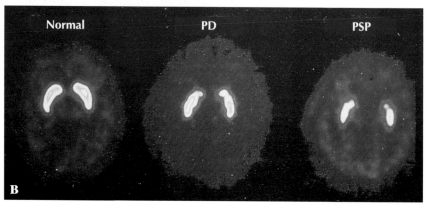

Table 2-6. Clinical Syndromes of Multiple System Atrophy

Shy-Drager Syndrome (SDS)

Parkinsonism (usually levodopa unresponsive)
Impotence (men)
Orthostatic hypotension
Labile blood pressure
Rectal incontinence
Fasciculations
Vocal cord paralysis with stridor

Olivopontocerebellar atrophy (OPCA)

Parkinsonism (usually levodopa unresponsive)
Ataxia
Nystagmus
Oculomotor disturbances
Facial dystonia in response to levodopa

Striatonigral degeneration (SND)

Parkinsonism (levodopa unresponsive)
Early falling
Corticospinal tract signs
Severe neck flexion
Vocal cord paralysis with stridor

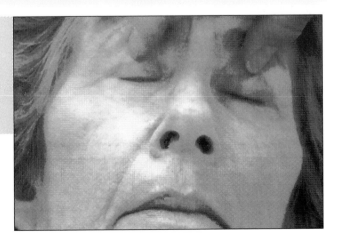

FIGURE 2-25 Reflex blepharospasm. This phenomenon is present in many types of parkinsonisms, including advanced Parkinson's disease. This patient has the striatonigral degeneration type of multiple system atrophy.

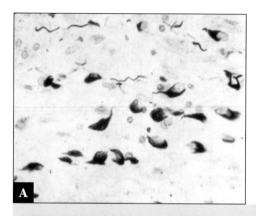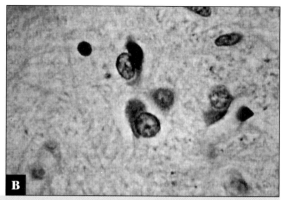

FIGURE 2-26 Cytoplasmic inclusion. **A**, Under low power, cytoplasmic inclusions and abnormal cell processes are seen (Gallyas silver staining). **B**, With higher power, ubiquitin-stained inclusions are seen in oligodendroglia in multiple system atrophy. (*From* Lantos and colleague (16); with permission.)

involvement of the putamen should be detectable in SND by neuroimaging techniques. Some reports have described decreased T2-signal on MRI in the putamen and decreased striatal glucose metabolism in patients with the SND variant of MSA (Figs. 2-27–2-30).

Cortical-Basal Ganglionic Degeneration

Clinical Characteristics

Cortical-basal ganglionic degeneration (CBGD) was first described in 1968 by Rebeiz and colleagues [17], who called it "cortico-dentato-nigral degeneration with neuronal achromasia" after the characteristic pathology. The disease was considered rare and not diagnosable during life, until several unique features were recognized. To date, over 60 cases have been reported, most without pathologic verification, so that the full spectrum of the condition is not certain. Typical patients present with markedly asymmetric parkinsonism and cortical deficits. One limb, usually the upper, but occasionally the lower, develops loss of dexterity, followed by athetotic posturing that progresses to dystonia, and then to a fixed posture that is sometimes painful. The cortical deficits include ideomotor apraxia, ideational apraxia, loss of graphesthesia or stereognosis, cortical focal myoclonus, and aphasia. The affected limb may have complex, unsuppressible movements, reminiscent of the "alien limb" phenomenon. Some patients have had prominent pseudobulbar palsy, with snout, palmomental, and grasp reflexes and emotional incontinence. There is a characteristic speech disturbance in which volume is preserved but

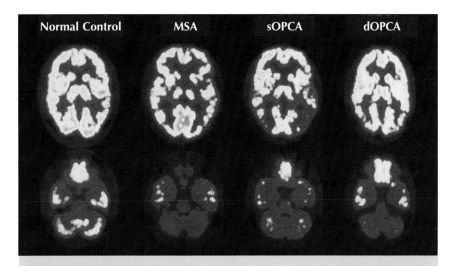

FIGURE 2-27 ^{18}F-Fluorodeoxyglucose positron emission tomography (PET) scans comparing a normal control; a patient with multiple system atrophy (MSA) who has parkinsonism, cerebellar, and autonomic dysfunction; a patient with sporadic olivopontocerebellar atrophy (sOPCA) who has parkinsonism and cerebellar dysfunction; and a patient with dominantly inherited OPCA (dOPCA) with cerebellar dysfunction. There is decreased cerebral metabolism in the cerebellum in the patient with MSA and in the patients with sOPCA and dOPCA. The cerebral cortex and basal ganglia have decreased glucose metabolism in MSA and sOPCA, but not in dOPCA. (*From* Gilman and colleagues (18); with permission.) (*See* Color Plate.)

speech becomes slurred and labored. Because of the speech and motor disturbances, communication becomes difficult. Although some patients have developed cognitive impairment, dementia has not been an early feature in most patients. Postural reflexes are lost early, and falling is an early feature of the condition. Supranuclear palsy may occur late in the course, and other disturbances of eye movement, characterized as apraxias, have been described. Occasionally, apraxia of eyelid opening and lower motor neuron signs have been reported. CBGD progresses more rapidly than PD, with a mean survival time of about 4 to 7 years after onset of symptoms (Fig. 2-31).

Pathology

The pathology of CBGD is characterized by cell loss, depigmentation, and gliosis in the substantia nigra with few, if any, Lewy bodies. There is also asymmetric cell loss and gliosis in focal areas of the cerebral cortex. Involvement of other subcortical areas is more variable, and the dentate nucleus is not invariably involved. There may be involvement of the putamen, globus

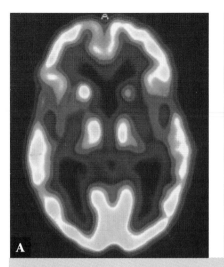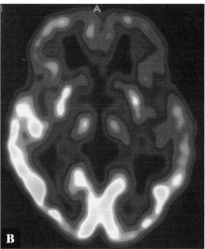

FIGURE 2-28 Fluorodeoxyglucose positron emission tomography (PET) scans in a patient with striatonigral degenerative (SND) compared to a patient with progressive supranuclear palsy (PSP). **A,** Striatonigral degeneration. **B,** PSP. Glucose metabolism is bilaterally reduced in the basal ganglia of the SND patient, more pronounced on the left. In the PSP patient, there is bilateral hypometabolism of basal ganglia, the thalamus, and particularly the orbito-frontal region. (*See* Color Plate.)

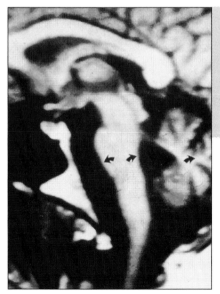

FIGURE 2-29 Magnetic resonance imaging (MRI) of a patient with olivopontocerebellar atrophy. The sagittal T1-weighted MRI demonstrates atrophy of the pons, brachium, and cerebellum (*arrows*). (*From* Rutledge and colleagues (19); with permission.)

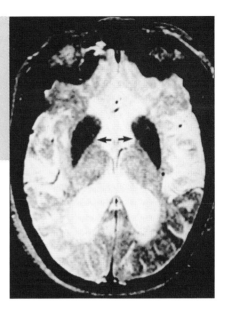

FIGURE 2-30 Transverse T2-weighted magnetic resonance image of a patient with striatonigral degeneration. The MRI demonstrates decreased signal intensity in the neostriatum (*arrows*), indicating increased iron deposition. (*From* Rutledge and colleagues (19); with permission.)

pallidus, caudate, thalamus, dentate, and subthalamus. The characteristic histologic findings are ballooned, poorly staining (achromatic) neurons in any of the above areas. These are similar, and may be identical, to abnormal cells found in Pick's disease, and a possible relationship between the two conditions has been suggested. New staining techniques have revealed cytoskeletal abnormalities in cortical neurons of patients with CBGD that may be unique to this disease (Figs. 2-32 and 2-33).

Hemiparkinsonism, Hemiatrophy Syndrome

In 1981, Klawans first identified patients with Parkinson symptoms limited to one side of the body and atrophy of the same side of the body (hemiparkinsonism/hemiatrophy syndrome [HP/HA]) [20]. These patients were younger at onset of disease than most patients with PD, tended to progress slowly, and symptoms remained limited to one side of the body. In subsequent reports, some patients with HP/HA have developed bilateral symptoms, but symptoms often remain strikingly asymmetric. Many have had dystonia of the affected side prior to taking anti-Parkinson therapy. The extent of atrophy is variable: some patients have hemiatrophy of the face and upper and lower extremities, whereas others

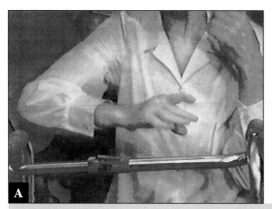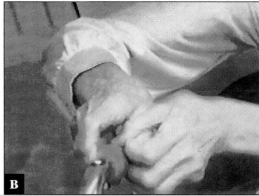

FIGURE 2-31 Unilateral dystonic and rigid right arm and hand in a patient with cortical-basal ganglionic degeneration. **A**, The patient has difficulty moving the right arm to the location she desires. **B**, To place or remove the apractic right hand onto or off of the handle of the walker, the patient needs to guide it with her left hand.

may have atrophy limited to one limb. Contralateral brain hemiatrophy may or may not accompany body hemiatrophy. Some patients have a history of birth injury, suggesting possible asymmetric damage to the substantia nigra early in life. The response to levodopa in HP/HA has ranged from poor to excellent (Fig. 2-34).

Parkinsonism-Dementia Syndromes

The common problem of parkinsonism and severe dementia presents a diagnostic challenge. Some dementia syndromes may include an akinetic-rigid state (*eg*, Creutzfeldt-Jakob disease, Pick's disease, Parkinson–dementia–amyotrophic lateral sclerosis complex of Guam), but account for a only a small percentage of patients with parkinsonism and severe dementia. Concurrent Alzheimer's disease probably accounts for a larger percentage of patients in this category, as patients with PD are believed to have an increased risk of developing Alzheimer's disease. More recently, it has been noted that some patients with parkinsonism and dementia (or dementia alone) will have a "diffuse Lewy body disease" (DLBD) when examined pathologically, with Lewy bodies in the neocortex and limbic regions in addition to the substantia nigra and other regions typical of Parkinson's disease. These patients were found to have a high prevalence of psychiatric symptoms (including agitation, hallucinations, and delusions), and tended to develop dementia before parkinsonism. The prevalence of DLBD is unknown (Fig. 2-35).

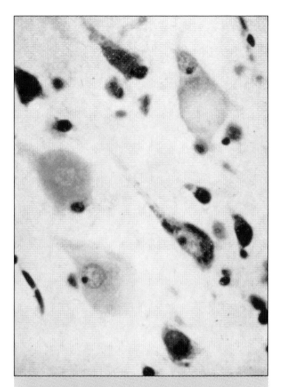

FIGURE 2-32 Achromatic, ballooned neuron with eccentric nuclei in cortical-basal ganglionic degeneration (cresyl violet stain, magnification x 650). (*From* Rebeiz and colleagues (17); with permission.)

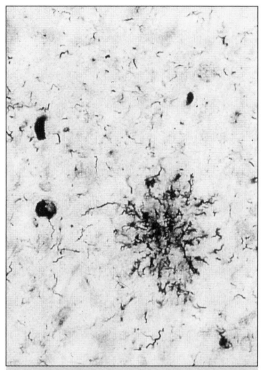

FIGURE 2-33 Cytoskeletal abnormalities in cortical-basal ganglionic degeneration (CBGD). The cytoplasm of the pyramidal neurons in the precentral cortex is densely stained. Star-like tufts and thread-like structures are visible (modified Gallyas stain, magnification x 300). (*From* Uchihara and colleagues (21); with permission.)

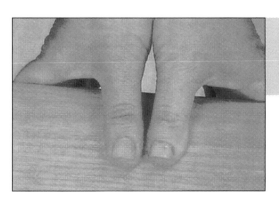

FIGURE 2-34 Patient with hemiparkinsonism/hemiatrophy, demonstrating the smaller-sized left thumb compared with the right.

Normal-pressure Hydrocephalus

In 1965, Hakim and Adams [22] described patients with gait disturbance, dementia, and urinary incontinence due to communicating hydrocephalus (large ventricles) with normal cerebrospinal fluid (CSF) pressure [22]. In some patients, trauma or subarachnoid hemorrhage preceded the development of symptoms, but in others there was no apparent cause. Patients with this condition of normal-pressure hydrocephalus (NPH) may improve temporarily after lumbar puncture, and may improve permanently after surgical diversion of CSF (eg, after ventriculoperitoneal shunting). Some patients with NPH seem to have their feet stuck to the ground, producing a "magnetic" gait, but other forms of gait disorder have also been observed. Patients with NPH may have facial masking, hypophonia, or other features of mild parkinsonism; thus NPH should be considered whenever gait disturbance is out of proportion to the other signs of parkinsonism. Enlarged ventricles and gait disorder, however, are not pathognomonic of NPH, and some patients with this combination do not improve after shunting. Some clinicians have used improvement after multiple daily lumbar punctures to identify patients who are candidates for surgical shunting. Attempts to find other radiologic or laboratory criteria for identifying patients who will improve after shunting have not been successful (Fig. 2-36).

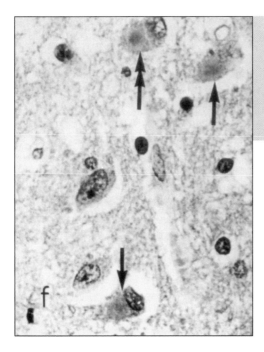

FIGURE 2-35 Cortical Lewy bodies (*arrows*) in a specimen from a patient with diffuse Lewy body disease. (*From* Perry and colleagues (23); with permission.)

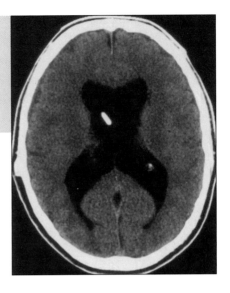

FIGURE 2-36 Computed tomography scan demonstrating the dilated ventricles of a patient with normal-pressure hydrocephalus. The patient had an excellent clinical response to ventriculopleural shunting.

References

1. Hughes AJ, Daniel SE, Kilford L, Lees AJ: Accuracy of clinical diagnosis of idiopathic Parkinson's disease: a clinico-pathological study of 100 cases. *J Neurol Neurosurg Psychiatr* 1992, 55:181–184.

2. Duvoisin RC, Eldridge R, Williams A, *et al.*: Twin study of Parkinson disease. *Neurology* 1981, 31:77–80.

3. Wichmann T, DeLong MR: Pathophysiology of parkinsonian motor abnormalities. *Adv Neurol* 1993, 60:53–61.

4. Polymeropoulos MH, Lavedan C, Leroy E, *et al.*: Mutation in the α-synuclein gene identified in families with Parkinson's disease. *Science* 1997, 276:2045–2047.

5. Lazzarini AM, Myers RH, Zimmerman TR, *et al.*: A clinical genetic study of Parkinson's disease: evidence for dominant transmission. *Neurology* 1994, 44:499–506.

6. Steele RC, Richardson JC, Olszewski J: Progressive supranuclear palsy: a heterogeneous degeneration involving the brain stem, basal ganglia and cerebellum with vertical gaze and pseudobulbar palsy, nuchal dystonia and dementia. *Arch Neurol* 1964, 10:333–359.

7. Chase TN, Mouradian NN, Engber TM: Motor response complications and the function of striatal efferent systems. *Neurology* 1993, 43(suppl 6):S23–S27.

8. Mouradian MM, Juncos JL, Fabbrini G, *et al.*: Motor fluctuations in Parkinson's disease: central pathophysiological mechanisms, part II. *Ann Neurol* 1988, 24:372–378.

9. Laitinen LV, Bergenheim AT, Hariz MI: Leksell's posteroventral pallido-tomy in the treatment of Parkinson's disease. *J Neurosurg* 1992, 76:53–61.

10. Lepore FE, Duvoisin RC: "Apraxia" of eyelid opening: an involuntary levator inhibition. *Neurology* 1985, 35:423–427.

11. Kordower JH, Freeman TB, Snow BJ, *et al.*: Neuropathological evidence of graft survival and striatal reinnervation after the transplantation of fetal mesencephalic tissue in a patient with Parkinson's disease. *N Engl J Med* 1995, 332:1118–1124.

12. Lantos PL: The neuropathology of progressive supranuclear palsy. In *Progressive Supranuclear Palsy: Diagnosis, Pathology and Therapy*. Edited by Tolosa E, Duvoisin R, Cruz-Sanchez FF. New York: Springer-Verlag, Wien 1994:137–152.

13. Graham JG, Oppenheimer DR: Orthostatic hypotension and nicotinic sensitivity in a case of multiple system atrophy. *J Neurol Neurosurg Psychiatry* 1969, 32:28–34.

14. Jellinger KA, Bancher C: Neuropathology. In *Progressive Supranuclear Palsy: Clinical and Research Approaches*. Edited by Litvan I, Agid Y. Oxford: Oxford University Press, 1992.

15. Brooks DJ: Pet studies in progressive supranuclear palsy. In *Progressive Supranuclear Palsy: Diagnosis, Pathology, and Therapy*. Edited by Tolosa E, Duvoisin R, Cruz-Sanchez FF. New York: Springer-Verlag: 1994:119–132.

16. Lantos PL, Papp MI: Cellular pathology of multiple system atrophy: a review. *J Neurol Neurosurg Psychiatry* 1994, 57:129–133.

17. Rebeiz JJ, Kolodny EH, Richardson EP Jr: Corticodentatonigral degeneration with neuronal achromasia. *Arch Neurol* 1968, 18:20–33.

18. Gilman S, Koeppe RA, Junck L, *et al.*: Patterns of cerebral glucose metabolism detected with positron emission tomography differ in multiple system atrophy and olivoponto-cerebellar atrophy. *Ann Neurol* 1994, 36:166–175.

19. Rutledge JN, Schallert T, Hall S: Magnetic resonance imaging in parkinsonisms. *Adv Neurol* 1993, 60:529–534.

20. Klawans HL: Hemiparkinsonism as a late complication of hemiatrophy: a new syndrome. *Neurology* 1981, 31:625–628.

21. Uchihara T, Mitani K, Mori H, *et al.*: Abnormal cytoskeletal pathology peculiar to corticobasal degeneration is different from that of Alzheimer's disease or progressive supranuclear palsy. *Acta Neurolpathol* 1994, 88:379–383.

22. Hakim S, Adams RD: The special clinical problem of symptomatic hydrocephalus with normal cerebrospinal fluid pressure: observations on cerebrospinal fluid hydrodynamics. *J Neurol Sci* 1965, 2:307–327.

23. Perry RH, Irving D, Blessed G, *et al.*: Senile dementia of Lewy body type. *J Neurol Sci* 1990, 95:119–139.

DYSTONIA

- ◆ Clinical Characteristics

- ◆ Electrophysiology

- ◆ Pathology

- ◆ Primary Dystonia

- ◆ Secondary Dystonias

- ◆ Treatment

Clinical Characteristics

Dystonia is defined as a syndrome of sustained muscle contractions, frequently causing twisting and repetitive movements or abnormal postures. The phenomenology of dystonic movements is varied, but certain features characterize dystonia and help distinguish it from other movement disorders:

1. The speed of contractions may be slow or rapid, and at the peak of movement, the contraction tends to be sustained.
2. Whatever the speed, contractions almost always have a consistent directional or patterned character; also they are predictably present in the affected muscle groups.
3. Dystonic contractions are usually aggravated during voluntary movement (action dystonia) and may only be present with specific actions such as writing.

The sustained, directional, patterned qualities of the movements distinguish dystonia from the simple shocklike contractions of myoclonus; the random, flowing, unsustained contractions characteristic of chorea; and the regular oscillations of tremor, although rhythmic dystonic tremor is not uncommon (Figs. 3-1 and 3-2).

One characteristic and almost unique feature of dystonia present in many patients, is the sensory trick or "geste antagoniste." Sensory tricks consist of tactile or proprioceptive maneuvers the patient performs that diminish dystonic movements. For example, patients with torticollis will often place their hand on the chin, side of the face, or occiput to reduce nuchal contractions; patients with oromandibular dystonia may obtain relief by placing an object such as a toothpick in the mouth; and patients with writer's cramp will often touch the affected hand with the other hand. The physiologic basis of sensory tricks is unknown (Figs. 3-3–3-5).

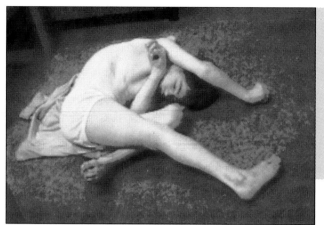

FIGURE 3-1 A patient with advanced childhood-onset generalized idiopathic torsion dystonia. This boy, who uses a wheelchair, is most comfortable lying on the floor in this position. The left hip, knee, elbow, and wrist are flexed; the right hip is flexed and the knee extended, the right arm is elevated with the elbow and wrist extended.

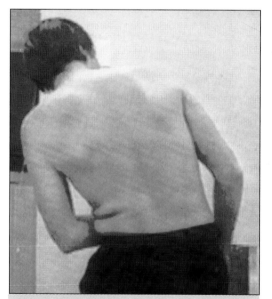

FIGURE 3-2 Scoliosis due to truncal dystonia.

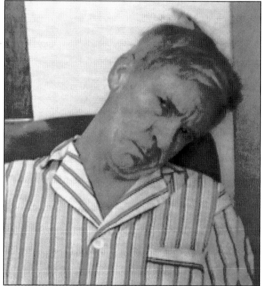

FIGURE 3-3 Severe cervical dystonia with the head tilted to the left in a sustained posture.

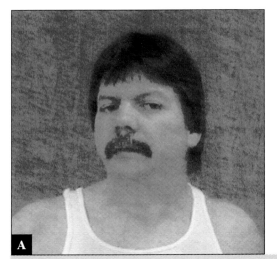
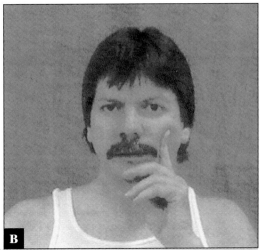

FIGURE 3-4   Patient with cervical dystonia (torticollis) **(A)** who has a lessening of the dystonia using a sensory trick **(B)**.

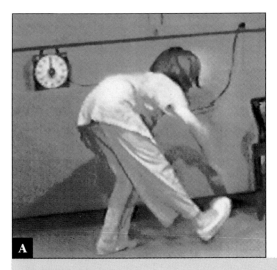
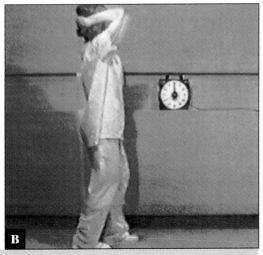

FIGURE 3-5   Patient with generalized dystonia **(A)** who has a lessening of the axial dystonia using a sensory trick **(B)**, namely placing a hand on the back of her head.

Dystonia is classified in three ways: by age at onset, body regions affected, and cause (Table 3-1). Clinical and genetic studies have shown that there is a strong relationship between the age at onset, which parts of the body are first affected, the progression or spread of dystonia to other body parts, and the cause [1]. Primary dystonia that begins in childhood and adolescence (early onset) usually first involves a leg or arm, and then spreads to other limbs and the trunk within 5 years. Most childhood-onset dystonia is due to mutations in a gene located on chromosome 9q34 [2]. This locus is called *DYT1*. Adult or late-onset primary dystonia usually starts in the neck, cranial muscles (including the vocal cords) (Figs. 3-8–3-9), or arm (Figs. 3-6–3-7); progression is limited and usually restricted to adjacent muscles. Leg involvement is very rare in adult-onset

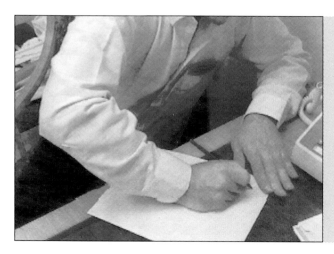

FIGURE 3-6

Writer's cramp, a focal dystonia of the arm induced with the action of writing. Note the elevation of the elbow off the surface of the desk by the dystonia of the proximal muscles of the arm.

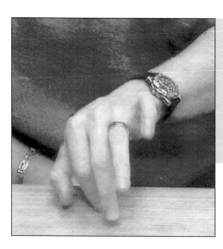

FIGURE 3-7 Musician's cramp, analogous to writer's cramp, is a focal dystonia of the arm induced with the action of playing a musical instrument. This patient has a pianist's cramp that is manifested when she attempts to perform piano-playing movements on top of the desk.

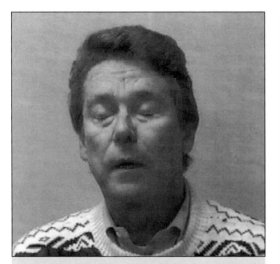

| FIGURE 3-8 | Blepharospasm. Involuntary closure of the eyelids. |

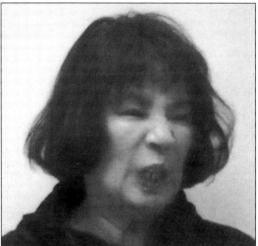

| FIGURE 3-9 | Cranial segmental dystonia, sometimes called Meige syndrome, with involvement of the facial and jaw muscles, and sometimes spreading to the neck muscles (cranial-cervical dystonia). |

primary dystonia, and this finding should raise the possibility that the leg dystonia is secondary to another disorder, such as Parkinson's disease. Similarly childhood-onset dystonia that begins in the cranial muscles is rare and again raises the issue that dystonia may be secondary or may represent another condition such as dystonic tics (see Table 3-1).

Electrophysiology

Dystonic movements at rest and with activity are characterized by a pattern of co-contraction of agonist and antagonist muscles. At rest there may be little or no activity or, in more severe cases, there may be one or more of three types of electromyogram (EMG) patterns: 1) long spasms that produce sustained postures; 2) repetitive, sometimes rhythmic, bursts of activity lasting 200 to 500 ms; and 3) irregular, brief (<100 ms) jerks resembling myoclonus. During voluntary movement all three types of EMG activity may occur. Typically, patients have difficulty selectively activating the appropriate muscles and have co-contraction of antagonists; also there is spread to muscles not normally involved (overflow). An abnormality detected in dystonia, which is related to the co-contraction described previously, is a decrease in reciprocal inhibition. Normally there is active inhibition in antagonist muscles during voluntary contraction of the agonist; this inhibition consists of an early phase of inhibition probably produced by spinal Ia inhibitory interneurons and a later, longer-lasting phase of inhibition produced by presynaptic inhibition on Ia afferent fibers. In dystonia there is a decrease in the amount of inhibition in the presynaptic (second) phase (Fig. 3-10).

Pathology

There is no consistent identified pathology in primary dystonia; however, many anatomic studies implicate the basal ganglia (and rarely, the brain stem) in secondary dystonia. Lesions have been found in the 1) striatum (both lentiform and caudate lesions producing limb or neck dystonia); 2) cortex (producing dystonia of the limbs, torticollis, or Meige's syndrome); 3) thalamus (producing limb dystonia, blepharospasm, or paroxysmal kinesigenic dystonia); 4) brain stem (blepharospasm); 5) cerebellum (torticollis); and 6) cervical cord (torticollis) (Fig. 3-11).

Table 3-1. Classification of Dystonia

Age at onset	Distribution	Cause
Early-onset (<21 years)	Focal (*eg*, writer's cramp, blepharospasm, torticollis, spasmodic dysphonia)	Primary (or idiopathic) dystonia is the only sign, and evaluation does not reveal an identifiable exogenous cause or other inherited or degenerative disease
Usually starts in a leg or arm and frequently progresses to involve other limbs and the trunk	Segmental (contiguous body regions involved; *eg*, face and jaw, arm and neck, both arms)	Secondary (or symptomatic)
Late-onset (>21 years)	Multifocal (non-contiguous body regions involved; *eg*, arm and leg, face, and arm)	Dystonia-Plus
Usually starts in the neck, cranial muscles, or arm and tends to remain localized with restricted spread to adjacent muscles	Generalized (both legs or one leg and trunk, and at least one other body region)	Presence of parkinsonism or myoclonus in addition to dystonia. Examples: dopa-responsive dystonia and dystonic myoclonus
		Heredodegenerative diseases
		Diseases such as Wilson's disease and Hallervorden-Spatz disease

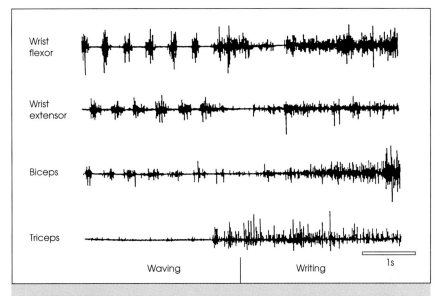

FIGURE 3-10 Normal reciprocal inhibition of wrist flexors and extensors during waving (*left*) and resumption of typical dystonic co-contraction when a patient with segmental arm dystonia stops to pick up a pen and write his name (*right*). This shows the abnormal co-contraction may only occur with specific actions, such as brachial dystonia that is elicited with writing but not other activities such as waving. (*From* Rothwell and colleagues (3); with permission.)

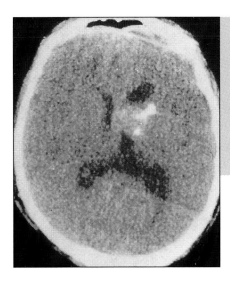

FIGURE 3-11 Computed tomography (CT) scan from a 38-year-old man with a 6-month history of left-turning torticollis. The scan shows a partially calcified enhancing lesion in the head of the right caudate nucleus that was found to be a venous angioma at operation. (*From* Marsden and colleagues (4); with permission.)

Primary Dystonia

Primary dystonia can develop at any age (Fig. 3-12). Early-onset dystonia (also known as dystonia musculorum deformans) represents about one ninth of all primary dystonias (Figs. 3-13). The prevalence of early-onset primary dystonia has been estimated to be between 1 to 4 per 100,000 in the non-Jewish population. It is about five times more common in Jews of Eastern European ancestry [5]; a recent study suggests an even higher prevalence of 30 per 100,000 in this population [6]. The disorder is inherited in an autosomal dominant fashion, with reduced penetrance of 30% to 40% [7]. Because of the low penetrance, and because relatives may have mild signs never diagnosed as dystonia, the patient is often the only one known to be affected in the family. The majority of early-onset cases are caused by the *DYT1* gene localized to chromosome 9q34 [2]. The *DYT1* gene mutation has been identified as a deletion of one of a pair of guanosine-adenosine–guanosine-trinucleotides in the gene that codes for the protein, torsin A [8]. In Ashkenazi Jews there is a strong association of a specific set of DNA markers that surrounds the *DYTI* gene causing early onset dystonia. This association indicates that dystonia in almost all early limb-onset Ashkenazi patients is due to a single "founder" mutation in the *DYT1* gene, and this mutation is estimated to be 350 years old [9]. The *DYT1* gene also underlies dystonia in most early-onset non-Jewish families studied for linkage to the *DYT1* locus; however, in these non-Jewish families, there is no evidence of an associated set of DNA markers to indicate a single founder mutation [2].

Late-onset dystonia represents eight ninths of primary dystonia cases (see Fig. 3-13). Its prevalence is estimated to be 29.5 per 100,000. Family studies of patients with late-onset focal dystonias indicate that at least some cases are inherited in an autosomal dominant fashion with reduced penetrance [6]. Linkage studies in a few large non-Jewish families with late-onset of symptoms [10] or prominent cranial and cervical involvement [11] have excluded the *DYT1* gene. At least one gene locus (*DYT7*) on chromosome 18 has been identified to underlie torticollis [12]. Another locus on chromosome 8 (*DYT6*) has recently been identified in Mennonite families with limb, cervical, and cranial dystonia [13].

Secondary Dystonias

Dystonia associated with inherited disease (approximately 5% of secondary cases) include dopa-responsive dystonia, myoclonic-dystonia, ataxia telangiectasia, Wilson's disease, Huntington's disease, spinocerebellar ataxias, GM_1 and GM_2 gangliosidoses, metachromatic leukodystrophy, Lesch-Nyhan syndrome, homocystinuria, glutaric acidemia, methylmalonic aciduria, triosephosphate isomerase deficiency, mitochondrial

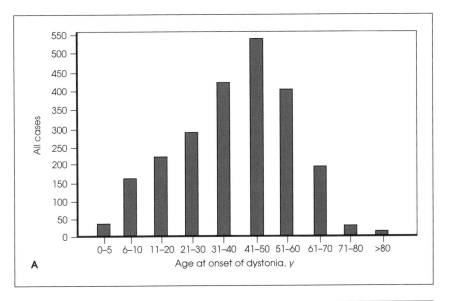

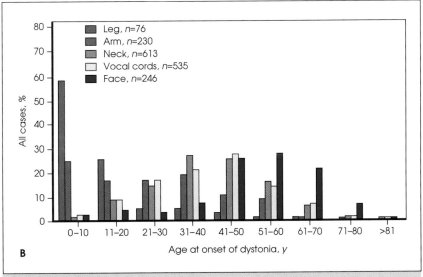

FIGURE 3-12   Age-at-onset distribution of primary dystonia. Age-at-onset distributions for (**A**) all cases, (**B**) for different sites at onset, and (*Continued*)

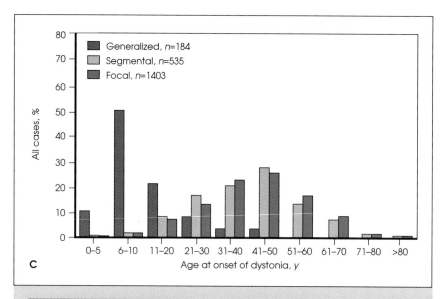

FIGURE 3-12 (continued) (C) for different distributions. The age-at-onset distributions of primary dystonia illustrate the different phenotypes observed in children and adults; the early-onset group consists primarily of limb-onset cases that frequently generalize; the late-onset group consists primarily of cervical and cranial-onset cases that remain localized as focal or segmental dystonia.

cytopathies, dentatorubropallidoluysian atrophy, neuroacanthocytosis, Hallervorden-Spatz disease, dystonic lipidoses, X-linked Dystonia-Parkinsonism, intranuclear hyaline inclusion disease, juvenile ceroid-lipofuscinosis, Fahr's disease (calcification of the basal ganglia), Rapid-onset Dystonia-Parkinsonism, Rett's syndrome, Pelizaeus-Merzbacher, and hereditary juvenile dystonia-parkinsonism (Fig. 3-14).

Diseases associated with degenerative disorders, and whose inherited basis has not been established (about 2% to 3% of secondary cases) include Parkinson's disease, progressive supranuclear palsy (PSP), cortical-basal ganglia degeneration (CBGD), and multiple system atrophy (MSA).

Diseases associated with environmental-exogenous factors (80% of secondary cases) comprise the largest group of secondary dystonia and include tardive dystonia due to dopamine receptor blockers (40%), perinatal cerebral anoxia, which may be delayed for years (15%), trauma (10%), stroke (cerebral infarction or hemorrhage) (5%), encephalitis (4%), tumor or vascular malformation (1%), and other conditions (5%). Psychogenic causes are associated with 13% of secondary dystonia cases.

One common cause of dystonia that is underestimated in tables of secondary causes of dystonia is Parkinson's disease (PD) and other parkinsonism disorders (PSP, MSA, CBGD). Although "pure" dystonia as a presenting sign of PD is not common, dystonic posturing, such as action-induced foot flexion, is a frequent early complaint. Further, trunk flexion

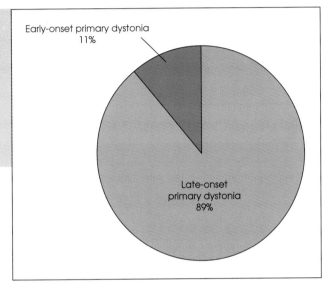

FIGURE 3-13 Proportions of all cases that are early- and late-onset dystonias. Early-onset represents one-ninth of the patients, and late-onset comprises eight-ninths of the total. (*Data from* the dystonia database of the Movement Disorder Group at Columbia-Presbyterian Medical Center's Dystonia Clinical Research Center.)

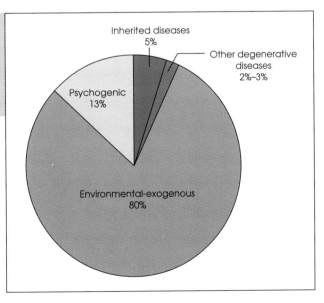

FIGURE 3-14 Causes for secondary dystonia in a movement disrorder clinic. About 30% of *all* dystonia in a movement disorder clinic is attributed to a secondary cause.

and tilt in the course of PD, and dystonia as a complication of levodopa therapy, are very common (Tables 3-2 and 3–3).

An outline of the diagnostic evaluation of patients with dystonia is presented in Figure 3-15.

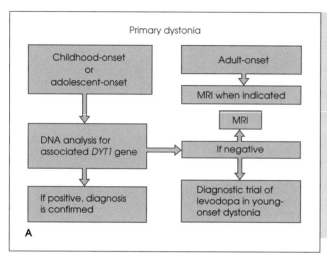

FIGURE 3-15 Diagnostic evaluation of dystonia. **A,** Primary dystonia. **B,** Secondary dystonia. ANA—antinuclear antibody; CSF—cerebrospinal fluid; CT—computed tomography; EEG—electroencephalogram; EMG—electromyogram; ERG—electroretinogram; ESR—erythrocyte sedimentation rate; MRI—magnetic resonance imaging; NCV—nerve conduction velocities; SMAC—serum chemistries including liver function tests; VLCFA—very long chain fatty acids.

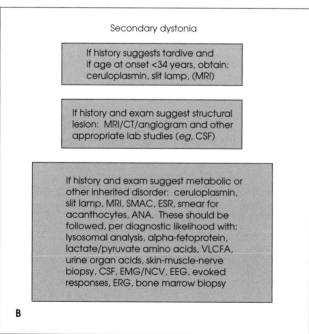

Table 3-2. Clinical Manifestations of Secondary Dystonia

History of a possible etiologic factor

Head trauma

Peripheral trauma

Encephalitis

Drug exposure

Toxin exposure

Perinatal anoxia

Presence of neurologic abnormality other than dystonia

Presence of false weakness, false sensory findings, or inconsistent or incongruous movements to suggest a psychogenic basis

Onset at rest rather than with action

Site of onset does not fit usual pattern seen in primary dystonia, such as cranial-onset in a child or leg-onset in an adult

Hemidystonia

Abnormal brain imaging

Abnormal laboratory work-up

Dopa-responsive Dystonia

Approximately 10% of patients with childhood-onset dystonia have dopa-responsive dystonia (DRD). This is an autosomal dominant condition, and penetrance is influenced by gender (females are more commonly affected). Many cases appear to be due to mutations in the gene for GTP cyclohydrolase 1; this is the first enzymatic step in the synthesis of tetrahydrobiopterin, a cofactor for tyrosine hydroxylase. Thus, partial deficiencies in this enzyme are thought to impair synthesis of dopamine [14] (Fig. 3-16).

Dopa-responsive dystonia mimics early-onset primary dystonia, with leg involvement and an abnormal gait being the first and predominant feature. Usually symptoms worsen as the day progresses and there may be improvement after a nap. The gait is frequently stiff-legged and there may be plantar flexion or eversion. Dystonia may also involve the trunk and arms, and less commonly the neck. Signs of parkinsonism are usually present but may be subtle; these include postural instability, hypomimia, and bradykinesia. There may be hyperreflexia, particularly in the legs, and plantar extensor signs; because of the hyperreflexia and the stiff-legged gait, children with DRD are often misdiagnosed as having spastic diplegic cerebral palsy [15]. The diagnosis of DRD depends on both the examination findings and a dramatic response to low dose levodopa. Treatment with as little as 50 to 200 mg of levodopa (together with a decarboxylase inhibitor) usually results in complete or near-complete reversal of all signs and symptoms. Further, patients do not develop fluctuations but maintain an excellent response to levodopa. In contrast, juvenile parkinsonism, which can begin with dystonia, requires higher doses of antiparkinson medication and typically is complicated by le-

Table 3-3. Clinical Signs Suggesting Secondary Dystonia

Parkinsonism	Neuropathy	Supranuclear oculomotor	Optic/Retinal	Ataxia
DRD	MLD	Dystonic-lipidoses	GM₂	Ataxia-telangiectasia
Wison's	Neuro-acanthocytosis	SCA1 and SCA3	HSD	Mitochondrial
Gangliosidosis	SCA1 and SCA3	Ataxia-telangiectasia	NCL	SCA1 and SCA3
HD	Mitochondrial	CBGD	Mitochondrial, including LHON	MLD
XPD		HD	Homocystinuria	Dystonic-lipidoses
RDP		Pallidal degeneration		NCL
HSD				Hartnup's
SCA3				Wilson's
Neuroacanthocytosis				
PD				
PSP				
CBGD				
Toxins: manganese, methanol, CS₂				
Anoxia				
Calcification of BG				
Hemiatrophy/hemiPD				

BG—basal ganglia; CBGD—cortical-basal ganglionic degeneration; CS₂—carbon disulfide; DRD—dopa-responsive dystonia; GM₂—gangliosidosis type 2; HD—Huntington's disease; HSD—Hallervorden-Spatz disease; LHON—Leber's hereditary optic atrophy; MJD—Machado-Joseph disease; MLD—metachromatic leukodystorphy; NCL—neuronal ceroid lipofuscinosis; PD—Parkinson's disease; PSP—Progressive supranuclear palsy; RDP—Rapid-onset dystonia parkinsonism; SCA1—spinocerebellar ataxia type 1; SCA3—spinocerebellar ataxia type 3; XPD—X-linked parkinsonism dystonia.

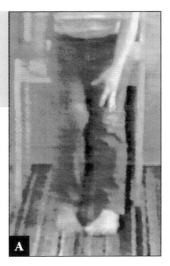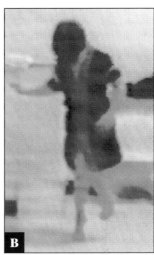

FIGURE 3-16 A patient with dopa-responsive dystonia, at the beginning of the day (**A**) and at the end of the day (**B**).

vodopa-related motor complications of dyskinesias and response fluctuations (Table 3-4).

Wilson's Disease

Because of the need for early recognition and treatment, Wilson's disease remains the most important diagnosis to consider when evaluating a patient with dystonia. Patients with neurologic Wilson's disease have Kayser-Fleischer (KF) rings (Fig. 3-17). The rings consist of yellow-brown deposits of copper in Descemet's membrane in the cornea and may only be visible through a slit lamp. Usually they are most dense at the upper and lower poles of the corneal limbus.

Signs of neurologic Wilson's usually manifest in the second or third decade, but may not be evident until the sixth decade. Dystonia, akinetic-rigid parkinsonism, and tremor with ataxia, titubation, and dysarthria are three common presenting syndromes. Drooling, risus sardonicus (a fixed grinning expression), clumsiness, and cognitive changes are usually present regardless of other signs. The responsible gene (a copper transporting P-type ATPase) for this autosomal recessive condition has been cloned [16,17] and over 20 different mutations in the gene have been identified [18]. Once a case is diagnosed, DNA analysis of linked markers can often be used to diagnose carrier status in a sibling, but direct DNA screening for mutations is not currently available. The diagnosis in a single patient, then, still depends on finding a reduced serum ceruloplasmin. About 5% of Wilson's patients have a normal ceruloplasmin level; thus diagnosis will depend on confirmatory evidence including KF rings, typical computed tomography (CT) and magnetic resonance imaging (MRI) changes, low serum copper, increased urine copper, and, if necessary, liver biopsy for copper content.

Hallervorden-Spatz Disease

This rare autosomal recessive disorder is characterized by dystonia, dysarthria, pyramidal signs, parkinsonism, dementia, and psychiatric symptoms. Pigmentary retinopathy or optic atrophy is seen in a significant proportion of patients. Onset is usually in childhood and adolescence, with progression to death by age 30; adult onset and a more slowly progressive course can, however, occur. Pathologically there is degeneration in the basal ganglia, especially the zona reticulata of the substantia nigra and the internal segment of the globus pallidus. These areas contain pigment-bound iron and axonal spheroids. The diagnosis is supported by MRI. Early on in the course of the disease there may be hyperintensity of the globus pallidus and substantia nigra on T3-weighted imaging; later these lesions become targetlike with a central area of hyperintensity surrounded by a hypointense ring. Another feature found in a subset of patients is acanthocytes on peripheral smear [19] (Fig. 3-18).

Striatal Lucencies and Dystonia

Striatal lucencies on CT scanning and T1-weighted MRI, or high-intensity signals on T3-weighted MRI, are seen in a number of conditions that produce dystonia. Causes for bilateral lesions include anoxia-ischemia, carbon monoxide poisoning, Wilson's disease, infantile striatal necrosis, and mitochondrial cytopathies, particularly Leigh's disease (Fig. 3-19).

Treatment

Because certain causes require specific treatments, the etiology must be assessed before initiating symptomatic treatment of dystonia. For example, Wilson's disease, acute drug-induced reactions, and tardive dystonia each call for a different treatment plan. One cause of dystonia, dopa-responsive dystonia (DRD), is *diagnosed by the response to treatment*. For the majority of patients, including all those with primary dystonia, as well as many patients with secondary forms of dystonia, symptomatic treatments can be ordered according to the distribution of muscle involvement.

Patients with early-onset generalized and segmental limb dystonia are treated first with levodopa; if there is no significant improvement after

Table 3-4. Differential Features Among Juvenile Parkinsonism, Dopa-responsive Dystonia and Childhood-onset Primary Early-onset Dystonia

	Juvenile parkinsonism	Dopa-responsive dystonia	Primary early-onset dystonia
Age-onset, y	8–21	Average 6, infancy to 12, rarely to 16	>4 and <44, average 9
Gender	Male > female	Female > male	Male = female
Initial sign	Foot dystonia	Leg dystonia	Limb dystonia
	Parkinsonism	Stiff-legged gait	Rarely neck or voice dystonia
Diurnal	No	Often	Rare
Bradykinesia	Yes	Yes	No
Postural instability	Yes	Yes	No
Initial response to levodopa	Yes with moderate or high dose	Yes with very low dose (25/100 mg)	None or slight
Long-term levodopa response	Fluctuations with dyskinesias	Stable	Unknown
Fluorodopa PET	Decreased	Normal or slightly decreased	Normal
CSF HVA	Decreased	Decreased	Normal
CSF biopterin	Moderately decreased	Markedly decreased	Normal
Gene	Unknown	GTP cyclohydrolase in many	DYT1 gene on 9q in most
Genetic testing	No	Research only	Commercial testing in Ashkenazi Jews
Prognosis	Progressive	Excellent with medication	Usually progresses at first, then plateaus

CSF—cerebrospinal fluid; GTP—guanosine triphosphate; HVA—homovanillic acid; PET—positron emission tomography.

slowly increasing to a daily dose of 300 mg of levodopa as carbidopa/levodopa, the diagnosis of DRD is excluded and other medications are then tried, beginning with anticholinergics. About 50% of patients will benefit to some degree with current medical therapies, but few are totally relieved of symptoms (Fig. 3-20).

For the majority of patients with focal dystonia, symptoms can be successfully ameliorated with botulinum toxin injections. About 90% of patients

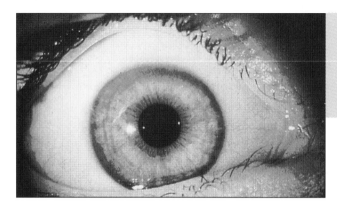

FIGURE 3-17 Early stage Kayser-Fleischer ring, located in the superior corneal pole only, in a patient with Wilson's disease. (*From* Wiebers and colleagues (20); with permission.)

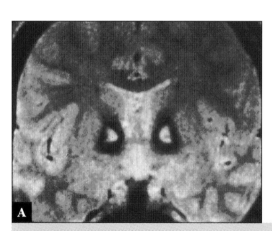
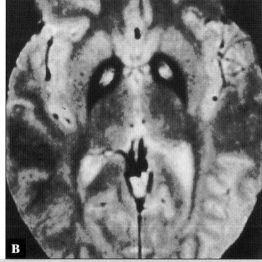

FIGURE 3-18 Magnetic resonance image of Hallervorden-Spatz disease depicting the "eye of the tiger" sign, in which the T3-weighted image shows a hyperintense signal (due to necrosis) surrounded by a hypointense signal (due to increased iron deposition) in the globus pallidus. **A**, Coronal view. **B**, Horizontal view. (*From* Sethi and colleagues (21); with permission.)

FIGURE 3-19 This magnetic resonance image is from a patient with a mitochondrial point mutation in the ND6 subunit of complex I. Clinical features of this disorder are dystonia (including the phenotype of childhood onset generalized dystonia with quadriparesis), Leber's hereditary optic neuropathy, or both. (*From* Shoffner and colleagues (22); with permission.)

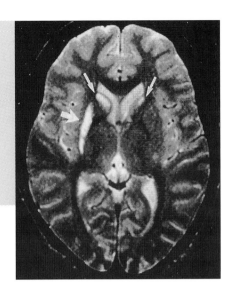

FIGURE 3-20 Treatment of dystonia. DRD—dopa-responsive dystonia.

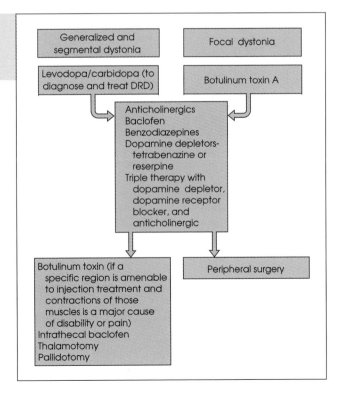

with blepharospasm and over 70% of patients with torticollis are moderately or markedly improved after botulinum toxin injections. Botulinum toxins are produced as fermentation products of the anaerobic bacterium *Clostridium botulinum*. Of the seven botulinum toxin (BTX) serotypes, BTX-A is the one most widely used in clinical practice. Injection of toxin into muscle causes temporary local muscle weakness by interfering with the release of acetylcholine from the presynaptic terminal at the neuromuscular junction.

References

1. Greene PE, Kang UJ, Fahn S: Spread of symptoms in idiopathic torsion dystonia. *Mov Disord* 1995, 10:143–152.
2. Kramer PL, Heiman GA, Gasser T, *et al.*: The DYT1 gene on 9q34 is responsible for most cases of early limb-onset idiopathic torsion dystonia in non-Jews. *Am J Hum Genet* 1994, 55:468–475.
3. Rothwell JC, Obeso JA, Day BL, Marsden CD: Pathophysiology of dystonias. In *Motor Control Mechanisms in Health and Disease*. Edited by Desmedt JE. New York: Raven Press, 1983:851–863.
4. Marsden CD, Obeso JA, Zarranz JJ, Lang AE: The anatomical basis of symptomatic hemidystonia. *Brain* 1985, 108:461–483.
5. Zilber N, Korcyn AD, Kahana E, *et al.*: Inheritance of idiopathic torsion dystonia among Jews. *J Med Genet* 1984, 21:13–26.
6. Waddy HM, Fletcher NA, Harding AE, Marsden CD: A genetic study of idiopathic focal dystonias. *Ann Neurol* 1991, 29:320–324.
7. Bressman SB, deLeon D, Brin MF, *et al.*: Idiopathic dystonia among Ashkenazi Jews: evidence for autosomal dominant inheritance. *Ann Neurol* 1989, 26:612–620.
8. Ozelius LJ, Hewett JW, Page CE, *et al.*: The early onset torsion dystonia gene (DYTI) encodes on ATP-binding protein. *Nat Genet* 1997, 17:40–48.
9. Risch N, De Leon D, Ozelius L, *et al.*: Genetic analysis of idiopathic torsion dystonia in Ashkenazi Jews and their recent descent from a small founder population. *Nat Genet* 1995, 9:152–159.
10. Holmgren G, Ozelius L, Forsgren L, *et al.*: Adult-onset idiopathic torsion dystonia is excluded from the DYT1 region (9q34) in a Swedish family. *J Neurol Neurosurg Psychiatry* 1995, 59:178–181.
11. Bressman SB, Hunt AL, Heiman GA, Brin MG, *et al.*: Exclusion of the DYT1 locus in a non-Jewish family with early-onset dystonia. *Mov Disord* 1994, 9:626–632.
12. Leube B, Rudnicki D, Ratzlaff T, *et al.*: Idiopathic torsion dystonia: assignment of a gene to chromosome 18p in a German family with adult onset, autosomal dominant inheritance and purely focal distribution. *Hum Mol Genet* 1996, 5:1673–1677.
13. Almasy L, Bressman SB, de Leon D, *et al.*: Idiopathic torsion dystonia linked to chromosome 8 markers in a family of German Mennonite origin. *Neurology* 1997, 48(suppl 2):A395.
14. Ichinose H, Ohye T, Takahashi E, *et al.*: Hereditary progressive dystonia

with marked diurnal fluctuation caused by mutations in the GTP cyclo-hydrolase I gene. *Nat Genet* 1994, 8:229–235.

15. Nygaard TG, Waran SP, Levine RA, *et al.*: Dopa-responsive dystonia simulating cerebral palsy. *Pediat Neurol* 1994, 11:236–240.

16. Bull PD, Thomas GR, Rommens JM, *et al.*: The Wilson disease gene is a putative copper transporting P-type ATPase similar to the Menkes gene [published erratum appears in *Nat Genet* 1994, 2:214]. *Nat Genet* 1993, 5:327–337.

17. Tanzi RE, Petrukhin K, Chernov I, *et al.*: The Wilson disease gene is a copper transporting ATPase with homology to the Menkes disease gene. *Nat Genet* 1993, 5:344–350.

18. Thomas GR, Forbes JR, Roberts EA, *et al.*: The Wilson disease gene: spectrum of mutations and their consequences. *Nat Genet* 1995, 9:210–217.

19. Higgins JJ, Patterson MC, Papadopoulos NM, *et al.*: Hypoprebetalipo-proteinemia, acanthocytosis, retinitis-pigmentosa, and pallidal degeneration (HARP syndrome). *Neurology* 1992, 42:194–198.

20. Wiebers DO, Hollenhorst RW, Goldstein NP: The opthalmologic manifestations of Wilson's disease. *Mayo Clin Proc* 1977, 52:409–416.

21. Sethi KD, Adams RJ, Loring DW, Gammal TE: Hallervorden-Spatz syndrome: clinical and magnetic resonance imaging correlations. *Ann Neurol* 1988, 24:692–694.

22. Shoffner JM, Brown MD, Stugard C, Jun AS, *et al.*: Leber's hereditary optic neuropathy plus dystonia is caused by a mitochondrial DNA point mutation. *Ann Neurol* 1995, 38:163–169.

Chapter 4

HUNTINGTON'S DISEASE AND OTHER CHOREAS

- ◆ Genetics

- ◆ Pathology and Imaging of Huntington's Disease

- ◆ Neuroacanthocytosis

- ◆ Sydenham's Chorea

- ◆ Dentatorubral-pallidoluysian Atrophy

Chorea refers to an irregular, nonrhythmic, rapid, unsustained involuntary movement that flows from one body part to another. Chorea is differentiated from other types of involuntary movements by its unpredictable quality. The timing, direction, and distribution are not patterned but random and changing. When infrequent, the brief, small amplitude movements of chorea can be difficult to distinguish from myoclonus. In Sydenham's and withdrawal emergent syndrome the movements may be very frequent and flowing, creating a picture of restlessness. Choreic movements can be partially suppressed and patients often camouflage the movements by incorporating them into semipurposeful movements, known as parakinesias. Chorea is also distinguished by the presence of motor impersistence (or negative chorea). A common symptom of impersistence is dropping objects; on examination impersistence is elicited by asking the patient to sustain a contraction, such as protruding the tongue or gripping the examiner's hand (impersistence of gripping is known as a "milk-maid" grip) (Fig. 4-1).

There are many causes of chorea and the long list of inherited disorders and exogenous factors that are associated with chorea presents a daunting diagnostic challenge for the clinician. However, the lengthy list of causes is somewhat misleading; many of them are apparent on history or produce other symptoms and signs that direct the order of work-up. The leading cause of adult-onset chorea is Huntington's disease. In children, infection and cardiac surgery are frequent causes. In all age groups, drug-induced chorea needs to be carefully investigated (Tables 4-1 and 4-2). Like other movement disorders, treatment of chorea needs to be tailored according to the etiology. Reduction of the choreic movements is often obtained with antidopaminergic medications, including dopamine depletors (eg, reserpine and tetrabenazine) and dopamine receptor blockers (eg, haloperidol, fluphenazine).

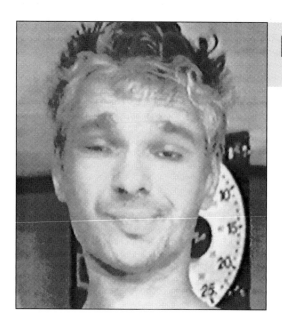

FIGURE 4-1 Facial choreic movements in a man with proven Huntington's disease.

Genetics

Huntington's disease (HD) is a true autosomal dominant condition, meaning that homozygotes and heterozygotes are clinically similar. The clinical features are presented in Table 4-2. The gene responsible for HD maps to chromosome 4p16.3 and codes a protein termed "huntingtin." Huntingtin is found in neurons throughout the brain but its function is unknown. The gene mutation in HD consists of an unstable expansion of a CAG repeat within the coding region of the gene that is translated into an expanded polyglutamine tract. The pathogenic mechanism of the enlarged polyglutamine stretch is not known but may involve the accumulation of an associated protein. Normal individuals and people with other diseases have about 20 CAG repeats (varying from six to 39); HD patients have over 35 (with a range from 35 to 121), with the vast majority having more than 39 repeats. A small number of asymptomatic individuals have "intermediate" sized repeats of 30-39. Their future development of HD and risk for transmitting a further expansion still needs to be assessed (Fig. 4-2) [1,2].

There is a negative correlation between the CAG repeat size in HD and the age at onset of symptoms. The correlation is most dramatic in the range of larger repeats and much less so in the shorter range; individuals with the same number of repeats may vary widely in their ages at onset. Furthermore, the repeat size does not determine the type of symptoms at onset. Because there is significant variation in disease expression that

Table 4-1. Major Causes of Chorea

Primary

Idiopathic
  Essential chorea
  Senile chorea
  Spontaneous oral dyskinesia
Hereditary
  Chorea is dominant feature
    Huntington's disease
    Hereditary nonprogressive
    chorea
    Neuroacanthocytosis

Chorea is not dominant
  feature
    Ataxia-telangiectasia
    Lesch-Nyhan syndrome
    Glutaric acidemia
    Cerebral lipidoses
    Familial chorea & myoclonus
    epilepsy
    Wilson's disease
    Pyruvate decarboxylase deficiency

Proprionic acidemia
Juvenile & adult GM_2
  gangliosidosis
Paroxysmal kinesigenic
  choreoathetosis
Paroxysmal nonkinesi-
  genic (dystonic)
  choreoathetosis

Secondary

Infectious
Sydenham's chorea
Encephalitides
Epidemic, SSPE, arthropod-borne,
  syphilis, measles, varicella, per-
  tussis, typhoid, mononucleosis,
  echovirus, AIDS,
  tuberculosis, Lyme disease
Subacute bacterial endocarditis
Creutzfeldt-Jakob disease
Typhoid fever
Immunologic
Systemic lupus erythematosus
Primary antiphospholipid anti-
  body syndrome
Paraneoplastic
Postvaccinal
Vascular
Hemichorea/hemiballism sec-
  ondary to stroke

Polycythemia vera
Henoch-Schönlein purpura
Internal cerebral vein thrombosis
Subdural hematoma
Chemicals/Toxins
Drugs
Levodopa, neuroleptics, anticholin-
  ergics, antihistamines, oral contra-
  ceptives, phenytoin, ethosuximide,
  imipramine, alpha methyldopa,
  methylphenidate, pemoline,
  methadone, cyproheptadine,
  cocaine
Chemicals: carbon monoxide, mer-
  cury, lithium, azide
Kernicterus
Alcoholism (hepatic?)
Metabolic and endocrine disorders
Chorea gravidarum
Birth control pills

Idiopathic hypoparathy-
  roidism
Hypomagnesemia
Addison's disease
Hypernatremia
Thyrotoxicosis
Hypoglycemia
Nonketotic hyper-
  glycemia
Chronic hepatocerebral
  degeneration
Anoxic encephalopathy
Mitochondrial
  cytopathies
Tumors including
  metastases
Multiple sclerosis
Tuberous sclerosis
Degeneration of cen-
  trum medianum

SSPE—subacute sclerosing panencephalitis.

cannot be explained by repeat size, great caution needs to be exercised in clinical interpretation of an expanded repeat other than predicting the eventual emergence of HD signs. One exception is in patients with very large repeats (>80). These are almost always associated with onset in adolescence or childhood and are usually paternally inherited. The explanation for the paternal excess of juvenile cases is that CAG repeats enlarge from generation

Table 4-2. Clinical Characteristics of Huntington's Disease

Age at onset

Childhood–80s (peaks in 4th or 5th decade)

Duration of illness

15–20 years for adult onset

10 years for juvenile onset

Chorea

Upper and lower facial

Limb and trunk

Motor impersistence (negative chorea)

Other neurologic signs

Abnormal saccades

Clumsy fine motor movements

Dancing or lurching gait

Postural instability

Dysarthria with abnormal rhythm
and slurring

Dysphagia

Dystonia

Tics (including noisy tics)

Ataxia*

Bradykinesia*

Rigidity*

Myoclonus*

Seizures*

Psychiatric signs

Apathy

Social withdrawal

Agitation

Impulsiveness

Hostility

Depression

Mania

Paranoia

Delusions

Hallucinations

Cognitive decline

Impaired attention

Impaired recent memory

Impaired judgment

Impaired psychomotor and executive function
(planning and initiation of activities and ability to switch from one plan to another)

Apraxia

Problems with verbal fluency

Especially likely to occur in those with juvenile onset before 20 years old.

to generation, but are more unstable and more likely to undergo a large expansion during male meiosis. A corollary of this instability in male meiosis is that "sporadic cases" or new mutations arise from expansions of paternal repeats in the intermediate range [3,4] (Figs. 4-3 and 4-4).

FIGURE 4-2 Number of CAG triplet repeats in 995 chromosomes affected with Huntington's disease (**A**) and 995 normal chromosomes (**B**). (*Adapted from* Kremer and colleagues (6); with permission.)

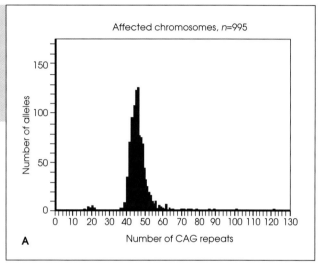

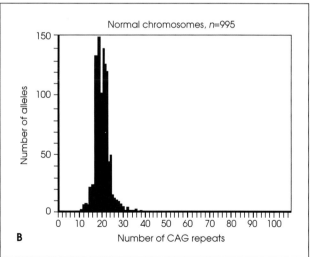

Pathology and Imaging of Huntington's Disease

The striatum bears the pathologic brunt in HD, although neuronal loss and gliosis also occur in the cortex. Medium-sized spiny neurons in the dorsomedial neostriatum, which project to the external pallidum and substantia nigra, degenerate first [5]. The selective loss of this subclass of GABA-ergic projection neurons is reproduced by intrastriatal injection of excitotoxic agonists of the *N*-methyl-*D*-aspartate (NMDA) receptor [7,8]. This experimental finding suggests an NMDA receptor or excitotoxic mechanism for HD (*eg*, a select group of striatal neurons may be vulnerable to the endogenous excitatory transmitter, glutamate). How the expanded huntingtin protein, which is expressed throughout the brain, produces selective vulnerability is not known.

Clinically, the selective pathology in HD is evidenced by computed tomography (CT), which shows caudate atrophy; magnetic resonance imaging (MRI) may be more sensitive, showing a reduction in the volume of the putamen before obvious caudate atrophy (Fig. 4-5). Glucose hypometabolism on positron emission tomography (PET) (Fig. 4-6) may also precede caudate atrophy on CT. None of these imaging techniques, however, reliably detects asymptomatic gene carriers, which requires DNA testing.

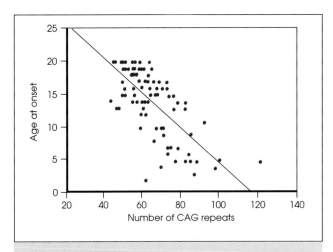

FIGURE 4-3 Negative correlation between CAG repeat size and age at onset of Huntington's disease. (*Adapted from* Bressman and colleague (9); with permission.)

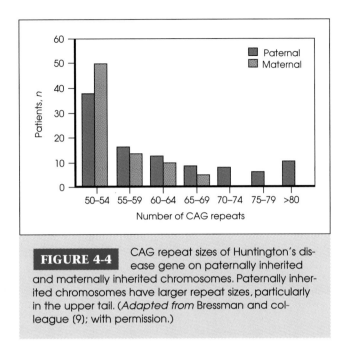

FIGURE 4-4 CAG repeat sizes of Huntington's disease gene on paternally inherited and maternally inherited chromosomes. Paternally inherited chromosomes have larger repeat sizes, particularly in the upper tail. (*Adapted from* Bressman and colleague (9); with permission.)

The selective loss of striatal GABA-ergic neurons that project to the external segment of the pallidum results in decreased inhibition of pallidal inhibitory efferents to the subthalamic nucleus (see Fig. 1-9); the subthalamic nucleus is then overinhibited, mimicking a subthalamic lesion. According to this model, the lack of subthalamic drive results in decreased output from the internal pallidum and thus less inhibition of the thalamus. The excessive thalamocortical drive to the premotor cortical regions results in chorea (Fig. 4-7).

Neuroacanthocytosis

The diagnosis of neuroacanthocytosis needs to be considered in patients with chorea, dystonia, tics, or parkinsonism. Symptoms usually begin in the third decade but there is a wide range of age onset—from 8 to 62 years. Typically there is lip and tongue biting that may be mutilating (Fig. 4-8) orolingual dystonia (with tongue protrusion) usually induced by eating, chorea, tics (including noisy smacking and hissing tics), parkinsonism, personality and cognitive changes, seizures, dysarthria, dysphagia, amyotrophy and areflexia. Laboratory findings include elevated creatine phosphokinase (CPK) and caudate atrophy on imaging studies. The diagnosis is made by finding that over 15% of erythrocytes are acanthocytes. Various techniques have been recommended to detect the acanthocytes, including diluting blood with normal saline, incubating a Wright-stained smear with EDTA, and using a scanning electron microscope [12]. The cause of neuroacanthocytosis is unknown but appears to be inherited. Pathologically there is neuronal loss in the striatum, pallidum, thalamus, nigra, and anterior horn cells. There are two other syndromes that overlap with neuroacanthocytosis: 1) the McLeod phenotype, which is an X-linked form of acanthocytosis associated with a particular erythrocyte Kell phenotype and clinical features of chorea, seizures, motor axonopathy, elevated CPK, hemolysis, and liver disease [13]; and 2) hypoprebeta-lipoproteinemia, acanthocytosis, retinitis pigmentosa, and pallidal degeneration (HARP syndrome), a form of Hallervorden-Spatz [14].

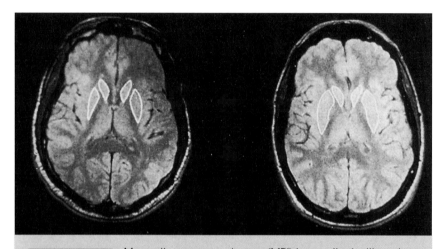

FIGURE 4-5 Magnetic resonance image (MRI) in a patient with early Huntington's disease (*left*) and a normal subject (*right*). In early Huntington's disease there is putaminal volume loss while the caudate nucleus appears normal. (*From* Harris and colleagues (10); with permission.)

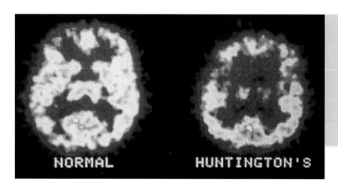

NORMAL   HUNTINGTON'S

FIGURE 4-6 A normal fluo-rodeoxyglucose positron emission tomography (PET) scan (*right*) and one showing Huntington's disease (*left*). In the PET scan on the left, striatal hypometabolism is seen. (*From* Martin and colleague (4); with permission.) (*See* Color Plate.)

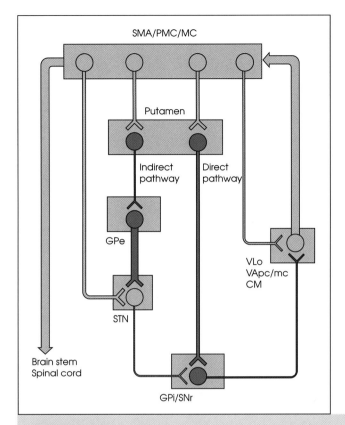

FIGURE 4-7 Pathophysiology of chorea. The net effect of the loss of GABA-ergic neurons of the "indirect" pathway in Huntington's disease is a net increase in inhibition of the subthalamic nucleus, analogous to mimicking a lesion of this nucleus. CM—centromedian nucleus of thalamus; GPe—globus pallidus externa; GPi—globus pallidus interna; MC—motor cortex; PMC—premotor cortex; SMA—supplementary motor area; SNr—substantia nigra pars reticulata; STN—subthalamic nucleus; VAmc—nucleus ventralis anterior pars magnocellularis; VApc—nucleus ventralis anterior pars parvocellularis; VLo—nucleus ventralis lateralis pars oralis. (*Adapted from* DeLong (11).)

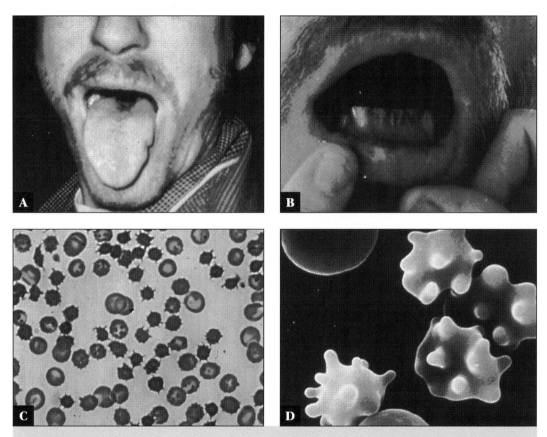

FIGURE 4-8 A 24-year-old man with neuroacanthocytosis and eating dystonia. He inflicted self-mutilations, which resulted in his biting off a piece of his tongue (**A**) and lip (**B**). A Wright-stained peripheral smear revealed acanthocytes (**C**) (*See* Color Plate.), which are also depicted on scanning electron microscopy (**D**).

Sydenham's Chorea

One cause of childhood chorea that is now less common due to the widespread use of antibiotics is Sydenham's chorea. Sydenham's chorea is considered a neurologic complication of group A streptococcus infection; pharyngitis may precede the onset of chorea by 1 to 6 months. Sydenham's may occur as a late aspect of the entire symptom complex of rheumatic fever (arthritis, carditis, rash) or may occur as the only manifestation. The chorea in Sydenham's differs somewhat from that in HD; it tends to be longer and has a more flowing quality. Although usually bilateral, chorea is often asymmetrical, and unilateral signs occur in about 20% of patients. Often there are behavioral disturbances (irritability, restlessness, attention deficit, obsessive-

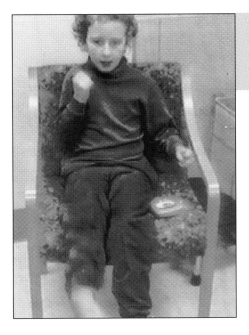

FIGURE 4-9 A child with hemiballism due to an astrocytoma involving the subthalamic nucleus.

compulsive symptoms), impersistence, and ataxia. More unusual associated features include dysarthria, confusion, cranial neuropathy, weakness, seizures, and headache. Sydenham's is self-limiting, usually lasting 3 to 4 months, but it can reappear with reinfection, pregnancy, or treatment with estrogen. The etiology is thought to be streptococcal-induced antibodies that crossreact with neuronal antigens in the caudate and subthalamic nucleus [15]. Interestingly, unlike other choreic disorders, PET scan indicates increased rather than decreased striatal glucose consumption [16]. Once the diagnosis is considered, an echocardiogram and electrocardiogram (EKG) need to be performed to evaluate possible cardiac involvement. Childhood choreic syndromes can be due to other causes also (Fig. 4-9).

Dentatorubral-pallidoluysian Atrophy

Dentatorubralpallidoluysian atrophy (DRPLA), like neuroacanthocytosis, is a condition that can mimic Huntington's disease. It was first described in 1946 and appears to be more common in Japan, although African American and European cases are described. The pathology is distinguished by involvement of the dentate nucleus and the external globus pallidus; the posterior columns may be involved also, and in one case this was the primary abnormality. The phenotype is quite varied and depends to some extent on the age at onset. Early-onset cases tend to show severe and rapid progression of myoclonus, epilepsy, and cognitive decline

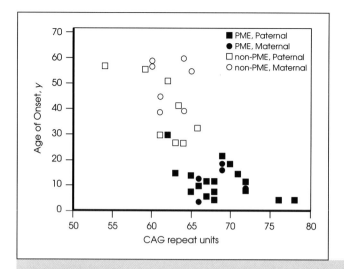

FIGURE 4-10 The correlation of CAG repeat size with age at onset, parental origins, and clinical phenotypes in patients with dentatorubralpallidoluysian atrophy (DRPLA). PME—progressive myoclonic epilepsy. (*Adapted from* Ikeuchi and colleagues (17); with permission.)

(myoclonic epilepsy), whereas late-onset cases display ataxia, chorea, and dementia and may be misdiagnosed as HD. Like HD, there is anticipation, and paternal transmission is associated with more severe, early-onset disease. Also like HD, the disorder is due to an unstable expansion of a CAG repeat in the coding region of the DRPLA gene, which maps to chromosome 12p. There is an inverse relationship between repeat size and age at onset, with controls having up to 26 repeats and disease alleles having 49 or more (Fig. 4-10). The gene is expressed in all tissues, including brain, and recent immunohistochemical studies indicate that the DRPLA gene product is observed mainly in neuronal cytoplasm [18]. The role of the polyglutamine stretch in the pathogenesis remains to be elucidated.

References

1. Huntington's Disease Collaborative Research Group: A novel gene containing a trinucleotide repeat that is expanded and unstable on Huntington's disease chromosomes. *Cell* 1993, 72:971–983.
2. Albin RL, Tagle DA: Genetics and molecular biology of Huntington's disease. *Trends Neurosci* 1995, 18:11–14.

3. Myers RH, MacDonald ME, Koroshetew J, *et al.*: De novo expansion of a (CAG)n repeat in sporadic Huntington's disease. *Nat Genet* 1993, 5:168–173.

4. Martin WRW, Calne DR: Imaging techniques and movement disorders. In *Movement Disorders* vol 2. Edited by Marsden CD, Fahn S. Boston: Butterworth; 1987:4–16.

5. Albin RL, Reiner A, Anderson KD, *et al.*: Preferential loss of striato-external pallidal projection neurons in presymptomatic Huntington's disease. *Ann Neurol* 1992, 31:425–430.

6. Kremer B, Goldberg P, Andrew SE, *et al.*: A worldwide study of the Huntington's disease mutation—the sensitivity and specificity of measuring CAG repeats. *N Engl J Med* 1994, 330:1401–1406.

7. Beal MF, Ferrante RJ, Swartz KJ, Kowall NW: Chronic quinolinic acid lesions in rats closely resemble Huntington's disease. *J Neurosci* 1991, 11:1649–1659.

8. Ferrante RJ, Kowall NW, Cipolloni PB, *et al.*: Excitotoxin lesions in primates as a model for Huntington's disease: histopathological and neurochemical characterization. *Exp Neurology* 1993, 119:46–71.

9. Bressman SB, Risch NJ: Genetics of movement disorders: dystonia, dopa-responsive dystonia and Huntington's disease. In *Movement and Allied Disorders*. Edited by Robertson MM, Eapen V. London: John Wiley and Sons; 1995, 327–356.

10. Harris GJ, Pearlson GD, Peyser CE, *et al.*: Putamen volume reduction on magnetic resonance imaging exceeds caudate changes in mild Huntington's disease. *Ann Neurol* 1992, 31:69–75.

11. DeLong MR: Primate models of movement disorders of basal ganglia origin. *Trends Neurosci* 1990, 13:281–285.

12. Feinberg TE, Cianci CD, Morrow JS, *et al.*: Diagnostic tests for choreoacanthocytosis. *Neurology* 1991, 41:1000–1006.

13. Witt TN, Danek A, Hein MU, *et al.*: McLeod syndrome: a distinct form of neuroacanthocytosis. *J Neurol* 1992, 239:302–306.

14. Orrell RW, Amrolia PJ, Heald A, *et al.*: Acanthocytosis, retinitis pigmentosa, and pallidal degeneration: a report of three patients, including the second reported case with hypoprebetalipoproteinemia (HARP syndrome). *Neurology* 1995, 45:487–491.

15. Husby G, Van de Rijn I, Zabriskie JB, *et al.*: Antibodies reacting with cytoplasm of subthalamic and caudate nuclei neurons in chorea and acute rheumatic fever. *J Exp Med* 1976, 144:1094–1100.

16. Weindl A, Kuwert T, Leenders KL, *et al.*: Increased striatal glucose consumption in Sydenham's chorea. *Mov Disord* 1993, 8:437–444.

17. Ikeuchi T, Koide R, Orodera O, *et al.*: Denatorubral-pallidoluysian atrophy (DRPLA). *Clin Neuroscience* 1995, 3:23–27.

18. Yazawa I, Nukina N, Hashida H, *et al.*: Abnormal gene product identified in hereditary dentatorubral pallidoluysian atrophy (DRPLA) brain. *Nat Genet* 1995, 10:99–103.

TICS

- ◆ Classification
- ◆ Treatment

Classification

Tics refer to spontaneous purposeless simple and complex movements or vocalizations that abruptly interrupt normal motor activity. There is often an associated sensation or urge to execute the tic and transient relief afterward. Tics are also temporarily suppressible. Typical tics include blinking, eye rolling, mouth opening, shoulder shrugging, head nodding, abdominal tensing, grunting, sniffing, and throat clearing. More complex tics include head shaking, trunk bending, kicking, and coprolalia.

Perhaps more than any other movement disorder, tics display the greatest range of phenomena and can resemble myoclonus, chorea, dystonia, or complex behaviors. A tic may consist of a fast (clonic), simple isolated jerk such as a blink, eye dart, or facial twitch; it may consist of a run of simple contractions such as repeated head nodding, shoulder shrugging or blinking. Alternatively the movement may be quite complex or sustained (*eg*, sustained eye deviation, jumping, copropraxia).

The great majority of tics are primary; 5% to 24% of school age children are estimated to have transient tics, and the prevalence of Tourette syndrome (TS) is estimated to be 30 to 40 per 100,000 (Table 5-1). For the diagnosis of TS both motor and vocal tics must be present for at least 1 year, and the age at onset must be under 21 years (mean age at onset is 7; 96% are affected by age 11). In TS, tics generally wax and wane in severity and one tic type is replaced by another; the tics usually begin in the face or neck (eyelid blinking and eyerolling are very common initial tics) but during the course of disease about half will involve the trunk or legs. Coprolalia, the most notorious sign in TS, is present in less than half of patients.

The etiologic (and specifically the genetic) relationship between TS, chronic tics, transient tics, and behavioral abnormalities (such as obses-

Table 5-1. Classification of Primary and Secondary Tics

Primary tics

Transient tic disorder
  (duration of tics <1 year)

Chronic multiple motor or vocal tics

Chronic single tic disorder

Tourette syndrome

Secondary tics

Infections
  Encephalitis
  Creutzfeldt-Jakob disease
  Sydenham's chorea
Drugs
  Stimulants
    Methylphenidate
    Amphetamines
    Cocaine
  Levodopa
  Anticonvulsants
  Antipsychotics (tardive tics)

Inherited disorders
  Huntington's disease
  Neuroacanthocytosis
Toxins
  Carbon monoxide poisoning
Perinatal injury
Other causes
  Head injury
  Chromosomal abnormalities
  Autistic disorders
  Mental retardation
  Stroke
  Neurocutaneous syndromes

sive compulsive disorder [OCD]) that occur with increased frequency in tic patients and their family members is debated. Some family studies [1] suggest that TS, chronic motor tics, and OCD are phenotypes of the same major gene that is inherited in an autosomal dominant fashion, with gender-influenced penetrance (it is higher in boys) and expression (girls are less likely to have TS and more likely to have OCD). Aside from OCD, other behavioral abnormalities that have been associated with tics include attention deficit hyperactivity, depression, anxiety, and conduct disorders. Although most investigators believe that at least some OCD is genetically related to TS, the etiologic relationship of other behavioral disorders to tics is controversial. A gene for TS has not been localized;

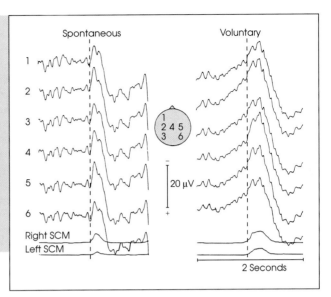

FIGURE 5-1 Recording of Bereitschaftspotential. Averaged electroencephalographic responses time-locked to muscle jerks in the right sternocleidomastoid muscle of a patient with Tourette syndrome. Records on the left are from spontaneous tics and show that the Bereitschaftspotential is not present. The tracing on the right records the patient mimicking the tics. The vertical dotted line indicates the start of the muscle jerk. SCM—sternocleidomastoid muscle. (*Adapted from* Obeso and colleagues (3); with permission.)

once it is, the phenotypic spectrum of TS can be more directly studied. The pathophysiology of TS is thought to involve a state of excess dopamine or hypersensitivity to dopamine. Dopamine receptors are not increased; however, dopamine hyperinnervation of the ventral striatum was suggested by one postmortem study [2].

One characteristic feature of tics that helps distinguish them from most other movement disorders is an associated urge to execute the tic or a more localized preceding sensory experience (*eg*, burning in the eyes before an eyeblink or roll, shoulder aching before a scapula rotation, or neck muscle tension before a head nod or jerk). Because of this associated sensory phenomena and the frequent relief of the sensation with tic execution, and also because tics can be transiently suppressed, patients often view their tics as intentional or semivoluntary. Electrophysiologic findings support the idea that tics are not normal voluntary actions; that is, normal planned voluntary movements are preceded on backaveraged electroencephalogram by a slow negative potential (the Bereitschaftspotential); as shown previously, these potentials are not observed before actual tics, but do occur when tics are voluntarily simulated (Fig. 5-1).

Treatment

Does a patient with tics need medical treatment? The decision to treat tics is based on the degree to which the abnormal movements and sounds disrupt the patient's daily function. The benefits of tic suppression must be weighed against the risk of any medication's adverse effects. A number of factors determine the severity of tics. Do tics interfere with school, work, social life? What is the major problem: tics, attention deficit, obsessions and compulsions?

Once it is decided to give medication, using a drug that does not produce a tardive dyskinesia syndrome, although usually less effective, is appropriate. If these fail, a dopamine receptor blocker may be necessary. For all drugs, start with a small dose and increase slowly, watching for side effects. Assure an adequate duration of drug trial on a sufficient dose before deciding on efficacy—tics wax and wane and it is difficult to separate therapeutic effect from the natural history in a single patient. Make changes as a sequence of single steps and always taper off slowly. This is especially true for dopamine receptor blockers—abrupt withdrawal can produce a withdrawal emergent syndrome (Table 5-2).

Table 5-2. Drugs Used to Treat Tic Disorders

Tics	Obsessive-compulsive disorder	Attention deficit disorder
Clonazepam	Imipramine	Clonidine
Clonidine	Fluoxetine	Imipramine
Baclofen	Sertraline	Desipramine
Tetrabenazine	Clomipramine	Selegiline
Risperidone	Clonazepam	Guanfacine
Fluphenazine	Carbamazepine	Methylphenidate
Pimozide		Pemoline
Haloperidol		
Trifluoperazine		
Thiothixene		
Botulinum toxin may be helpful for dystonic tics such as blinking/blepharospasm and neck jerks		

References

1. Pauls DL, Raymond CL, Stevenson JM, Leckman JF: A family study of Gilles de la Tourette syndrome. *Am J Human Genet* 1991, 48:154–163.
2. Singer HS, Hahn IH, Krowiak E, *et al*.: Tourette's syndrome: a neuro-chemical analysis of postmortem cortical brain tissue. *Ann Neurol* 1990, 27:443–446.
3. Obeso JA, Rothwell JC, Marsden CD: The neurophysiology of Tourette syndrome. *Adv Neurol* 1982, 35:105–114.

TREMOR

Tremor is a rhythmic oscillation of a body part that is produced by alternating or synchronous contractions of opposing muscles. Tremors may be classified on the basis of clinical appearance, distribution, etiology, or physiologic characteristics. Phenomenologically, tremors are classified according to two main categories: tremors at rest and tremors with action. Rest tremors occur when the affected body part is in complete repose and fully supported. The classical tremor of Parkinson's disease (PD) is a tremor at rest, but it tends to re-occur when the limbs are outstretched. The PD rest tremor may be easily observed when the patient is walking. Action tremors occur with voluntary muscle contractions and are subdivided into postural, kinetic, task- or position-specific, and isometric tremors. Postural tremors are observed in an outstretched limb maintained against gravity. Kinetic tremors occur during directed movement, such as reaching for an object or the finger-to-nose task of the neurologic exam. An action tremor that increases as the finger approaches the target is often termed a *terminal tremor*, or *intention tremor*, and suggests a clinical localization to the cerebellum or its outflow tracts. Task-specific tremors only occur during, or are greatly increased during, the performance of a coordinated task, such as writing or playing a musical instrument. Isometric tremors occur during voluntary muscle contraction that is not accompanied by any movement, such as during isometric exercises.

Tremor frequency may provide a clue as to tremor etiology. Two commonly observed tremors in clinical practice include essential tremor and the tremor of PD, usually in the 4 to 8 Hz range of frequency. Tremors accompanying diseases of the cerebellum or its outflow tracts often have a frequency in the range of 2 to 3 Hz. Physiologic tremors are faster, often in the range of 8 to 10 Hz.

The probable origin of the PD tremor is spontaneous bursting of neurons within the thalamus that drives the cortical neurons and is transmitted via the corticospinal tract to the motor neurons in the spinal cord. This neurophysiologic sequence of events occurs as a result of nigrostriatal dopamine depletion, leading to disinhibition of the subthalamic nucleus (Table 6-1).

Differential Diagnosis of Tremor

Tremor can be caused by a wide spectrum of neurologic and medical conditions. The differential diagnosis of tremor can be categorized into tremors at rest and action tremors. Table 6-2 presents these tremors in greater detail.

Physiologic Tremor

Physiologic tremor is the oscillation of a body part resulting from the interaction of normal mechanical reflex mechanisms and a central oscillator. The usual frequency of physiologic tremor ranges between 8 to 12 Hz. The frequency of the mechanical component of the physiologic tremor is influenced by mechanical properties of the oscillating limb, including stiffness and inertia. Tremor amplitude is determined by synchronization of motor unit discharges, and is enhanced under certain conditions such as anxiety, stress, fatigue, hypoglycemia, thyrotoxicosis, and pheochromocytoma. The frequency of physiologic tremor recorded at the wrist decreases with mass loading, a mechanical phenomenon that does not occur with essential tremor or the tremor of Parkinson's disease (Figs. 6-1 and 6-2) [1].

Normal physiologic tremor may become prominent under certain circumstances ("exaggerated physiologic tremor"), including conditions known to enhance the activity of peripheral β-adrenergic receptors, present in muscle fibers. The mechanisms producing exaggerated physiologic tremor may enhance all types of pathologic tremor.

Essential Tremor

Essential tremor (ET) may be the most prevalent of all movement disorders, affecting as many as 10% of individuals over age 65 [2]. Essential tremor is often regarded as a benign, nonprogressive neurologic condition, but the tremor may progress to the point of physical or social disability in some individuals. The true prevalence of essential tremor is hard to ascertain because most individuals have mild symptoms and do not present for medical evaluation. Moreover, there is controversy as to the diagnostic criteria for essential tremor. To date, there is no specific diagnostic test for essential tremor. Essential tremor may show variable electrophysiologic features, but the tremor frequency of essential tremor does not decrease with mass loading, differentiating this tremor from exagger-

Table 6-1. Etiology, Clinical, and Electrophysiologic Characteristics of Tremors

Type of tremor	Etiology	Clinical and electrophysiologic characteristics
Rest	Parkinson's disease	3 to 6 Hz tremor occurring at rest, suppressed by posture-holding or action. Often most prominent during walking. The rest tremor of Parkinson's disease not infrequently returns with prolonged posture-holding, giving a "re-emergent rest tremor."
Action, posture-holding	Exaggerated physiologic tremor	8 to 12 Hz tremor occurring with action and posture-holding, often induced by specific stress, precipitant, or medication. Tremor frequency is reduced by inertial loading.
Posture-holding and action	Essential tremor	Symmetric postural and kinetic tremor of the arms, usually in the 4 to 10 Hz range, due to co-contracting antagonists. Essential tremor can be brought out by the tasks of the neurologic examination. It may interfere with activities of daily living, including handwriting.
Action, posture-holding, and sometimes at rest	Midbrain tremor	Classically described as an intention tremor, or sometimes ataxic tremor, midbrain tremor can manifest as a combination of rest, postural, and action tremors. The tremor frequency is usually between 2 to 5 Hz. Commonly caused by a focal lesion in the midbrain affecting cerebellothalamic and nigrostriatal pathways due to trauma, stroke, hemorrhage, or multiple sclerosis.
Kinetic and posture-holding	Dystonia	Irregular, asynchronous tremor, usually affecting arms or neck. Dystonic tremor has no specific electrophysiologic characteristics, but the dystonia manifests as co-contracting antagonists. Tremor may decrease with sensory trick or assumption of a "null point" posture. Includes primary writing tremor and task-specific tremor.

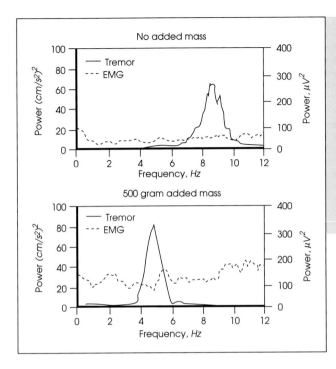

FIGURE 6-1 The frequency of physiologic tremor recorded at the wrist. Normal physiologic tremor may become prominent under certain circumstances ("exaggerated physiologic tremor"), including conditions known to enhance the activity of peripheral β-adrenergic receptors, present in muscle fibers. The mechanisms producing exaggerated physiologic tremor may enhance all types of pathologic tremor. EMG—electromyogram. (*From* Elble (1); with permission.)

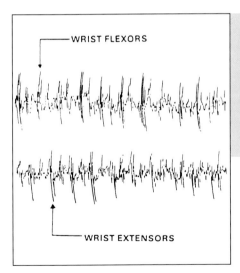

FIGURE 6-2 Electromyogram recordings of a forearm tremor in a patient at rest with MPTP-induced parkinsonism. The recording reveals alternating agonist and antagonist discharges bursting at approximately 5.5 Hz. (*From* Tetrud and colleague (3); with permission.)

ated physiologic tremor. Patients with essential tremor frequently report a positive family history, a reduction in tremor due to alcohol, and responsiveness to a β-blocker or primidone. However, these do not constitute diagnostic criteria for essential tremor. It is possible that genetic tests will be developed for the diagnosis of essential tremor, but these will not likely predict the time of onset, clinical severity, or course for gene carriers.

A proposed set of diagnostic criteria based on the clinical appearance of the tremor, categorizing essential tremor as definite, probable, or possible, is presented in Table 6-2 (Fig. 6-3).

Tremor in Parkinson's Disease

The tremor of Parkinson's disease is predominantly a 3 to 6 Hz tremor of the limb at rest. Typically, the tremor reduces or disappears when the affected limb is engaged in an activity or posture-holding. The tremor appears to result from central oscillatory activity in parts of the basal ganglia. In monkeys with experimental parkinsonism treated with the neurotoxin MPTP (l-methyl-4-phenyl-1,2,3,6-tetrahydropyridine), bursts of electrical spikes recorded in the subthalamic nucleus are synchronous with tremor oscillations observed in the contralateral limb [4] (Fig. 6-4, Table 6-3).

Thalamic Stimulation and Thalamotomy for Treatment of Tremor

All types of tremor can be abolished by electrical stimulation or by a lesion placed in the contralateral thalamic nucleus ventralis intermedius (Vim). Figure 6-5 shows a cross-section of the left thalamus in a patient with the rest tremor of Parkinson's disease who had been treated with an implanted stimulator. The tip of the stimulator produced a 3.5 mm gliotic lesion within the Vim nucleus (Fig. 6-6).

Midbrain Tremor

A paramedian infarction of the midbrain tegmentum produces a contralateral ataxia and intention tremor caused by damage in the red nucleus and brachium conjunctivum. *Claude syndrome* is a combination of midbrain tremor, ataxia, and ipsilateral third nerve palsy; the additional presence of contralateral corticospinal tract signs is *Benedikt syndrome* [5] (Fig. 6-7).

Table 6-2. Proposed Diagnostic Criteria for Essential Tremor

Criteria for definite essential tremor (ET) (all 5 must be true)

1. On examination, a +2 postural tremor of at least 1 arm. (A head tremor may also be present but is not sufficient for the diagnosis.)

2. On examination, there must be

a. a +2 kinetic tremor during at least 4 tasks, or

b. a +2 kinetic tremor on 1 task and a +3 kinetic tremor on a second task. Tasks include pouring water, using a spoon to drink water, drinking water, finger-to-nose movements, and drawing a spiral.

3. If on examination the tremor is present in the dominant hand, then by report, it must interfere with at least 1 activity of daily living (eating, drinking, writing, or using the hands). If on examination the tremor is not present in the dominant hand, then this criterion is irrelevant.

4. Medications, hyperthyroidism, alcohol, or dystonia are not potential etiologic factors.

5. Not psychogenic (eg, bizarre features, inconsistent in character, changing, distractable, or other psychiatric features on examination).

Criteria for probable ET (1, 3, 4, and 5 must be true. Also, either 2a or 2b must be true)

1. On examination, a +2 postural tremor of arms may or may not be present.

2a. Same as criterion 2 above (see definite ET).

2b. Head tremor is present on examination.

3. Tremor in the dominant hand may or may not interfere with at least 1 daily activity.

4. Medications, hyperthyroidism, dystonia, or alcohol are not potential etiologic factors.

5. Not psychogenic.

Criteria for possible ET

1. On examination, a +2 kinetic tremor must be present on 3 tasks.

2. No other stipulations.

Tremor ratings

0 = no visible tremor

+1 = low amplitude or barely perceivable tremor or intermittent tremor

+2 = tremor is of moderate amplitude (1–2 cm), usually present, and clearly oscillatory

+3 = large amplitude (>2 cm), violent, jerky tremor resulting in difficulty completing the task because of spilling or inability to hold a pen to paper

(From Louis and colleagues [4]; with permission.)

FIGURE 6-3 A man with essential tremor spilling water when he attempts to pour it from one cup to another.

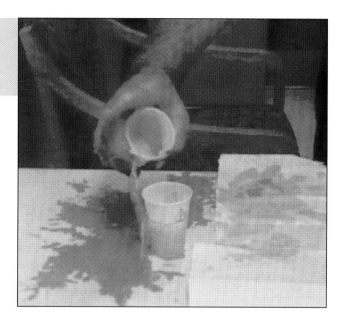

FIGURE 6-4 Parkinsonian tremor. Bursts of electrical spikes recorded in the subthalamic nucleus (**A**) of monkeys with parkinsonism who were treated with MPTP (1-methyl-4-phenyl-1,2,3,6-tetrahydropyridine) are synchronous with tremor oscillations observed in the contralateral limb (**B**). The tremor of Parkinson's disease is predominantly a 3 to 6 Hz tremor of the limb at rest. Typically, the tremor reduces or disappears when the affected limb is engaged in an activity or posture-holding. The tremor appears to result from central oscillatory activity in parts of the basal ganglia. A parkinsonian tremor can be abolished by a contralateral lesion in the thalamic nucleus ventralis intermedius (Vim) or by electrical stimulation of the nucleus. (*Adapted from* Vitek and colleagues (6).)

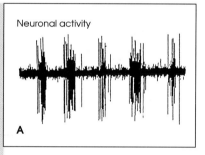

Neuronal activity

A

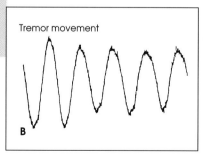

Tremor movement

B

Table 6-3. Parkinson's Disease Versus Essential Tremor

	Parkinson's disease	**Essential tremor**
Tremor	Occurs at rest Decreases with posture-holding or action Increases with walking	Posture-holding and action
Distribution	Asymmetrical, sometimes unilateral	Symmetrical
Body part	Hands, legs	Hands, head, voice
Drawing a spiral	Micrographic	Tremulous
Age at onset	Middle age or elderly	All ages
Course	Progressive	Stable or slowly progressive
First degree relatives	Usually unaffected	Often affected
Other neurologic signs	Bradykinesia, rigidity, postural instability	None
Substances that decrease tremor	Anticholinergics, levodopa	Alcohol, propranolol, primidone

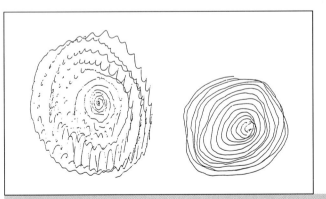

FIGURE 6-5 Spirals drawn by patients with essential tremor and Parkinson's disease tremor. Essential tremor can interfere with drawing a smooth spiral, as seen in the left panel. The patient with Parkinson's disease may have a tremor at rest that *decreases* upon action or writing; however, the spiral may be micrographic, as in the right panel. (*Courtesy of* Seth Pullman, MD, Columbia-Presbyterian Medical Center, New York, NY.)

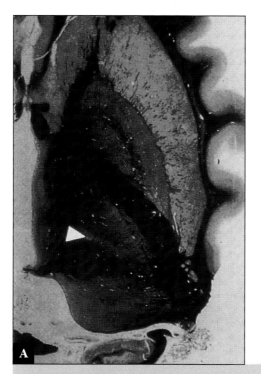

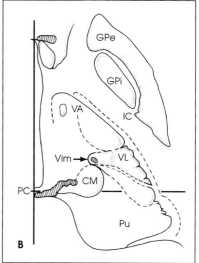

FIGURE 6-6 Cross-section of the left thalamus in a patient treated with an implanted stimulator. **A,** Brain section through the thalamus. **B,** Thalamic subdivisions. The position of the upper part of the stimulating electrode is indicated (*arrow*). CM—centromedian nucleus; Gpe—globus pallidus external segment; GPi—globus pallidus internal segment; IC—internal capsule; PC—posterior commisure; Pu—pulvinar; VA—ventral anterior nucleus; Vim—ventralis intermedius nucleus; VL—ventral lateral nucleus. (*From* Caparros-Lefebvre and colleagues (7); with permission.)

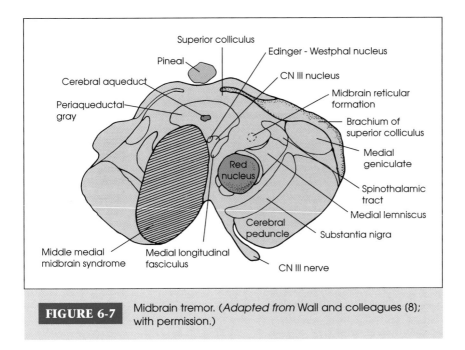

Superior colliculus
Edinger - Westphal nucleus
Pineal
CN III nucleus
Cerebral aqueduct
Midbrain reticular formation
Periaqueductal gray
Brachium of superior colliculus
Red nucleus
Medial geniculate
Spinothalamic tract
Medial lemniscus
Cerebral peduncle
Substantia nigra
Middle medial midbrain syndrome
Medial longitudinal fasciculus
CN III nerve

FIGURE 6-7   Midbrain tremor. (*Adapted from* Wall and colleagues (8); with permission.)

References

1. Elble RJ: Mechanisms of physiological tremor and relationship to essential tremor. *Handbook of Tremor Disorders*. Edited by Findley LJ, Koller WC. New York: Marcel Dekker, 1995; 51–62.
2. Louis ED, Marder K, Cote L, *et al.*: Prevalence of a history of shaking in persons 65 years of age or older: diagnostic and functional correlates. *Mov Disord* 1996, 11:63–69.
3. Tetrud JW, Langston JW: MPTP-induced Parkinsonism and Tremor. In *Handbook of Tremor Disorders*. Edited by Findley LJ, Koller WC. New York: Marcel Dekker; 1995; 51–62.
4. Louis ED, Ford B, Pullman SL: Prevalence of asymptomatic tremor in relatives of patients with essential tremor. *Arch Neurol* 1997, 54:197–200.
5. Bogousslavsky J, Maeder P, Regli F, Meuli R: Pure midbrain infarction: clinical syndromes, MRI, and etiologic patterns. *Neurology* 1994, 44:2032–2040.
6. Vitek JL, Wichmann T, DeLong MR: Current Concepts of Basal Ganglia Neurophysiology Relative to Tremorgenesis. In *Handbook of Tremor Disorders*. Edited by Findley LJ, Koller WC. New York: Marcel Dekker; 1995; 319–332.
7. Caparros-Lefebvre D, Ruchoux MM, Blond S, *et al.*: Long-term thalamic stimulation in Parkinson's disease. *Neurology* 1994, 44:1856–1860.
8. Wall M: Brainstem Syndromes. In *Neurology in Clinical Practice*. Edited by Bradley WG, Daroff RB, Fenichel GM, Marsden CD. Boston: Butterworth-Heinemann; 1991:347–362.

MYOCLONUS

◆ Progressive Myoclonic Epilepsy

◆ Myoclonus in Creutzfeldt-Jakob Disease

◆ Asterixis

◆ Treatment of Myoclonus

The term that describes brief, sudden, shock-like muscle contractions is *myoclonus*. Electrophysiologically, a myoclonic jerk is due to a brief electromyographic (EMG) burst of 10 to 50 msec, and rarely longer than 100 msec. Sudden, brief limb jerks may be caused not only by a quick forceful muscular contraction but also a sudden lapse of muscular contraction when the affected limb is maintained in a sustained posture, termed *negative myoclonus*, or *asterixis*. Myoclonic jerks may be repetitive and rhythmic or random and unpredictable. Myoclonus may represent a major or primary neurologic complaint, interfering with gait or coordination, or it may be a minor, even subtle, finding that is noted on examination by the careful observer. Myoclonus may occur at rest, with posture-holding or directed movement (action myoclonus), or be triggered by external stimulation (reflex myoclonus), whether auditory, tactile, or visual.

The diagnostic approach to myoclonus has a dual objective: identifying the site of the origin of myoclonus within the nervous system and establishing the cause. Myoclonus may be classified on the basis of its clinical characteristics, distribution (focal, segmental, multifocal, generalized), site of origin (cortical, brain stem, spinal cord, or peripheral nerve) (Fig. 7-1) or its etiology (Table 7-1). Synchronous myoclonic jerks affecting most of the body constitute *generalized myoclonus*. Myoclonus confined to a segment of the body, such as the shoulder girdle, is termed *segmental myoclonus*. *Multifocal myoclonus* describes myoclonic jerks widely distributed throughout the body, occurring often in an unpredictable and unsynchronized fashion (Table 7-2).

Myoclonus may be physiologic or pathologic. Myoclonus is a feature of several epilepsy syndromes, but can occur in a great number of other conditions, including degenerative, toxic, metabolic, vascular, traumatic, and others.

Cortical myoclonus originates in the sensorimotor cortex, and is propagated via the corticospinal tract. It may manifest as isolated muscle jerks,

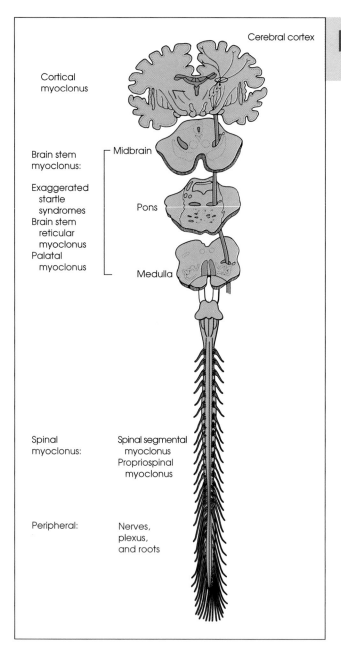

FIGURE 7-1 Localization of myoclonus. (*Adapted from* Carpenter (1).)

reflecting a restricted motor neuron pool. Repetitive focal myoclonic jerks may represent epilepsia partialis continua (continuous focal motor seizures). Focal myoclonic seizures may propagate, and become secondarily generalized.

Jerk-locked electromyography to electroencephalography back-averaging is a helpful electrophysiological technique in localizing myoclonus of a cortical origin. Routine electroencephalographic recordings often do not reveal an abnormal cortical discharge in relation to a myoclonic jerk (Figs. 7-2 and Fig. 7-3).

Somatosensory evoked potentials (SSEPs) are useful in the study of myoclonus. Giant SSEPs are often present in cortical myoclonus. The response consists of a characteristic waveform recorded from the cerebral cortex after an electrical stimulus is applied to a contralateral limb. The technique has consistently demonstrated giant SSEPs in patients with progressive myoclonic epilepsy, a syndrome that encompasses several rare disorders, including sialidosis, Lafora body disease, mitochondrial encephalomyopathy and ragged red fibers (MERRF), and neuronal ceroid lipofuscinosis (NCL). Most myoclonic disorders not in this disease category do not have giant SSEPs.

Myoclonus of brain stem origin may present as an exaggerated startle reflex or hyperekplexia, brain stem reticular myoclonus, or the palatal myoclonus syndrome. Two forms of spinal myoclonus are characterized: spinal segmental myoclonus, restricted to a few spinal segments, and propriospinal myoclonus, producing generalized axial jerks. Peripherally induced myoclonus arises from a lesion of the peripheral nervous system, including the spinal roots, plexus, or nerve; the best known example is hemifacial spasm caused by a lesion of the facial nerve.

Progressive Myoclonic Epilepsy

Progressive myoclonic epilepsy (PME) describes a syndrome that includes myoclonus and progressive neurologic decline usually ending in death. A severe seizure disorder, sometimes characterized by multiple types of seizures, may accompany the syndrome. The differential diagnosis of PME is dominated by several rare childhood-onset metabolic conditions, including sialidosis (cherry red spot myoclonus syndrome), mitochondrial encephalopathy (such as myoclonic epilepsy and ragged red fibers [MERRF], Lafora body disease, Unverricht-Lundborg disease, and neuronal ceroid lipofuscinosis (Table 7-3).

Table 7-1. Localization, Electrophysiology, Clinical Manifestations, and Etiology of Myoclonus

Localization and type	Electrophysiology
Cortical myoclonus	Abnormal activity originates in the sensorimotor cortex and is transmitted to the spinal cord by the corticospinal tract; diagnostic features may include large amplitude SSEPs and a cortical focus identified by jerk-locked EMG to EEG backaveraging
Brain stem	
Exaggerated startle syndromes, or hyperekplexia	Diffuse brain stem abnormality
Brain stem reticular myoclonus	Diffuse brain stem abnormality, utilizes pathways independent of startle reflex
Palatal myoclonus	Abnormal discharge due to brain stem pathology affecting dentato-olivary pathway in the central tegmental tract
Spinal cord	
Spinal segmental myoclonus	Abnormal discharge due to focal spinal cord pathology
Propriospinal myoclonus	Focal spinal cord generator, involves long propriospinal fibers distributed to axial musculature in an orderly sequence
Peripheral nerve	
Focal myoclonus	Generator presumed to be a peripheral nerve or root

EEG—electroencephalogram; EMG—electromyogram; SSEPs—somatosensory evoked potentials.

Clinical manifestations

Spontaneous muscle jerks, sometimes restricted to a body part, may have secondary generalization; jerks may be triggered by external stimuli (cortical reflex myoclonus) or may occur on movement (cortical action myoclonus)

Generalized axial jerks and other motor responses triggered by unexpected external stimuli

Generalized axial muscle jerks, beginning in the muscles of the lower brain stem, and spreading both rostrally and caudally

Rhythmic palatal movements at about 1.5 to 3 Hz, often accompanied by an audible click Myoclonus may persist during sleep

Jerking of a body part, sometimes rhythmic, involving a few spinal segments

Generalized axial jerks, usually beginning in abdominal muscles and spreading up and down the trunk

Focal myoclonic jerks restricted to a segment of the body, often a proximal limb, trunk musculature, or muscles innervated by the facial nerve (hemifacial spasm)

Etiology

Focal myoclonus may be due to a focal lesion in cerebral cortex (tumor, trauma, vascular lesion), focal epilepsy or epilepsia partialis continua

Multifocal or generalized myoclonus may be due to primary generalized epilepsy, progressive myoclonic epilepsy, encephalitis, Creutzfeldt-Jakob disease, Alzheimer's disease, degenerative disease, hypoxia, toxic states, and various metabolic encephalopathies

Local brain stem pathology (anoxia, multiple sclerosis), hereditary hyperekplexia

Cerebral anoxia, uremia, and other toxic or metabolic states

Focal brain stem lesion, usually due to stroke, multiple sclerosis, tumor, or trauma

Focal lesion, such as trauma, tumor, multiple sclerosis, vascular lesion

Focal lesion occasionally found

Focal neurovascular lesion, nerve compression, trauma, demyelination, radiation injury

Table 7-2. Etiologic Classification of Myoclonus

Physiologic myoclonus
Sleep jerks (hypnic myoclonus)
Hiccup (singultus)
Benign infantile myoclonus

Essential myoclonus
Unknown cause, no other neurologic abnormality
Hereditary
Sporadic

Epileptic myoclonus: *clinical syndrome dominated by seizures*
Infantile myoclonus
Lennox-Gastaut syndrome
Myoclonic absences
Epilepsia partialis continua
Juvenile myoclonic epilepsy

Progressive myoclonic epilepsy: *clinical syndrome dominated by progressive encephalopathy*
Mitochondrial encephalopathy—myoclonic epilepsy and ragged red fibers (MERFF)
Ramsay-Hunt syndrome
Lafora body disease
Sialidosis
Neuronal ceroid lipofuscinosis
Unverricht-Lundborg disease

Symptomatic causes of myoclonus
Trauma
Creutzfeldt-Jakob disease
Viral encephalopathy—subacute sclerosis panencephalitis (SSPE)
Degenerative disease—Alzheimer's disease, Parkinson's disease, atypical parkinsonism
Metabolic encephalopathy—hepatic failure, renal failure
Toxic encephalopathy—bismuth, heavy metals
Post-hypoxic
Brain tumor
Stroke

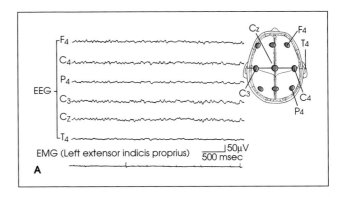

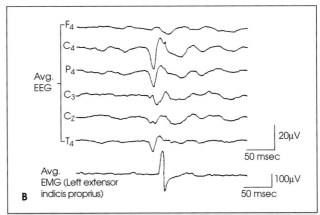

FIGURE 7-2 Cortical myoclonus. **A,** Electroencephalographic (EEG) recording with simultaneous electromyographic (EMG) activity from the left extensor indicis proprius (index finger muscle). No paroxysmal electroencephalographic activity is seen despite the frequent miniature myoclonic jerks recorded from the electromyogram. **B,** Averaged recording of 100 samples of electroencephalographic activity, each triggered by the electromyographic pulse of a single myoclonic jerk, and demonstrating an obvious biphasic spike over the right central hemisphere in close temporal relation to the electromyographic discharge. (*Adapted from* Shibasaki and colleague (2).)

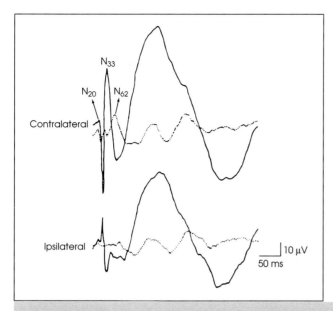

FIGURE 7-3 Giant somatosensory-evoked potentials (SSEPs) in progressive myoclonic epilepsy. SSEPs are useful in the study of myoclonus. The response consists of a characteristic waveform recorded from the cerebral cortex after an electrical stimulus is applied to a contralateral limb.

In this diagram, the SSEP is recorded following an electrical stimulation of the median nerve just proximal to the wrist in a patient with progressive myoclonic epilepsy. The dotted tracing represents the normal response. The negative (upward) deflections are labeled N20, N33, and N62, corresponding to the time in milliseconds following the electrical stimulus. In the patient with myoclonus, the N33 peak has a mean amplitude of 41 ´V, approximately 17 times larger than normal. The technique has consistently demonstrated giant SSEPs in patients with progressive myoclonic epilepsy, a syndrome that encompasses several rare disorders, including sialidosis, Lafora body disease, mitochondiral encephalomyopathy and ragged red fibers (MERRF), and neuronal ceroid lipofuscinosis (NCL). Most myoclonic disorders not in this disease category do not have giant SSEPs. (*Adapted from* Shibasaki and colleagues (3); with permission.)

Myoclonus in Creutzfeldt-Jakob Disease

Creutzfeldt-Jakob disease (CJD) is a rare, fatal, transmissible encephalopathy characterized clinically by a rapidly progressive dementia and myoclonus. The electroencephalogram (EEG) reveals a characteristic pattern of periodic sharp wave complexes. In Figure 7-4, periodic complexes in a patient with CJD predominate over the left hemisphere, corresponding to rhythmic myoclonic jerks of the right arm. The electrooculogram (EOG) records abrupt ocular deviations to the left, in synchrony with the periodic complexes and limb myoclonus.

Asterixis

Asterixis is characterized by sudden brief lapses of sustained posture. Asterixis can be demonstrated by having the patient extend the arms and dorsiflex the hands in a sustained posture (Fig. 7-5). Electrophysiologically, asterixis consists of abrupt, brief periods of EMG silence, usually lasting 50 to 200 msec, occurring against a background of tonic muscle contraction (Fig. 7-6).

Similarities between asterixis and myoclonus have lead to the concept that asterixis is a form of negative myoclonus [4]. The main clinical significance of asterixis is its frequent association with a toxic or metabolic encephalopathy. The typical clinical setting is uremia, hepatic encephalopathy, electrolyte imbalance, hypercarbia, hypoxia, anticonvulsant treatment, sedative use, or a similar condition. Associated features in a patient with asterixis generally include a depressed level of consciousness and slowing of the EEG. Negative myoclonus generally proves more resistant to treatment.

Treatment of Myoclonus

A number of drugs may be helpful in the treatment of myoclonic jerks. Clonazepam and valproate are usually the most effective. A systematic trial of the drugs in Table 7-4 is often necessary.

Table 7-3. Progressive Myoclonic Epilepsies

Progressive myoclonic epilepsy	Usual age at onset, y	Clinical features	Diagnosis	Age at death
Neuronal ceroid lipofuscinosis Infantile (Haltia-Santavuori) [Chromosome 1 p32]	0–2	Blindness, ataxia, hypotonia, developmental regression	Biopsy (electron microscopy) of skin, rectal mucosa, brain: Lysosomal lipopigment storage, curvilinear granular inclusions, fingerprint bodies PAS and cytoplasmic inclusion bodies in skin, muscle, liver, and brain biopsy	Infancy
				Childhood
				20 years (Batten's disease)
Late infantile (Bielschowsky-Jansky)	2–4	Seizures, ataxia, spasticity, dementia		10 years after onset
Juvenile Batten's disease, Spielmeyer-Vogt [Chromosome 16 p12]	4–10	Visual loss, mild ataxia, slowly progressive dementia, personality change		
Adult (Kufs)	11–50	Ataxia, spasticity, rigidity, chorea		
Lafora disease [Chromosome 6]	10–18	Blindness, dementia	PAS and Lafora bodies (polyglycosans) in sweat glands, muscle, liver, brain	10 years after onset
Mitochondrial encephalomyopathy with ragged red fibers (MERRF)	3–65	Myopathy, ataxia, myoclonic, epilepsy, short stature	Muscle biopsy: Ragged fibers respiratory chain metabolic deficit, mtDNA mutation 8344	3-30 years after onset
Sialidosis (Cherry red spot myoclonus) Type I [chromosome 20] Type II [chromosome 10 pter-p23, chromosome 22]	8–15	Dementia, spasticity, facial myoclonus, burning paresthesias, ataxia	Increased urinary oligosaccharides; fibroblasts and lymphocytes: α-n-acetyl neuraminidase deficit	10-40 years after onset

Gaucher's disease [Chromosome 1 p21]	5-15	Gaze palsy, splenomegaly, bone pain, spasticity, dementia, ataxia	Increased acid phosphatase, β-glucocerebroside β-glucocerebrosidase activity decreased in fibroblasts or lymphocytes, Gaucher cells and increased glucocerebroside in lymphocytes, bone marrow	
Unverricht-Lundborg disease (Baltic myoclonus, Mediterranean myoclonus) [Chromosome 21q.22.3]	6-15	Mild cognitive impairment	Vesicular changes in eccrine sweat glands No specific marker	50-60 years
Dentatorubropalli-doluysian atrophy (DRPLA) [Chromosome 12p]	Childhood–adulthood	Chorea, dementia	DNA triplicate repeats CAG	
Juvenile GM$_2$ gangliosidosis (Type II) [Chromosome 15]	2-6	Ataxia, dementia, visual loss, corticospinal tract signs, retinitis pigmentosa	Leukocyte β-N-acetylhex-osaminidase A deficiency	Adulthood 5-15 years

PAS—periodic acid-Schiff. (Adapted from Delgado-Escuota and colleagues [5]; with permission.)

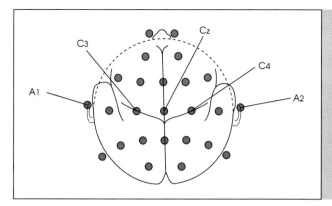

FIGURE 7-4 Electroencephalogram (EEG) and electrooculogram (EOG) in a patient with Creutzfeldt-Jakob disease. In this EEG periodic sharp wave complexes predominate over the left hemisphere, corresponding to rhythmic myoclonic jerks of the right arm. The EOG records abrupt ocular deviations to the left, in synchrony with the periodic complexes and limb myoclonus. (*From* Shibasaki and colleagues (6); with permission.)

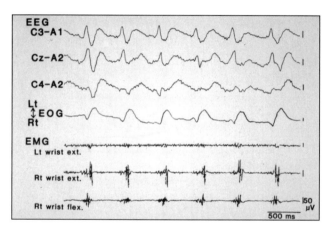

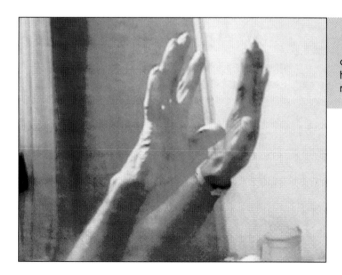

FIGURE 7-5 Testing for asterixis. The patient dorsiflexes the wrists to allow the hands to "flap" when the extensor muscles are suddenly inhibited.

FIGURE 7-6 Electromyographic tracing of forearm extensor activity using surface electrodes, with time callibrations of 250 ms, in a patient with asterixis. The arrows denote a period of electrical silence, corresponding to negative myoclonic jerks, or asterixis. (*Adapted from* Young and colleague (7); with permission.)

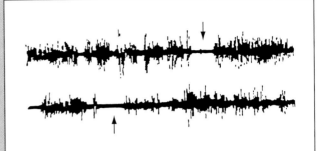

Table 7-4. Treatment of Myoclonus

Medication	Dose range	Indication
ACTH	150 units/m²/d	Infantile spasms, opsoclonus
Clonazepam	0.5 to 20 mg/d	Most forms of myoclonus
5-hydroxytryptophan	25 mg qid to 500 mg qid	Posthypoxic myoclonus
Piracetam	400 mg tid to 16 g/d	Cortical myoclonus
Tetrabenazine	25 mg/d to 300 mg/d	Segmental myoclonus
Valproic acid	15 mg/kd/d to 2000 mg/d	Most forms of myoclonus

ACTH—adenocorticotropic hormone.

References

1. Carpenter MB: *Core Text of Neuroanatomy*, edn 3. Baltimore: Williams & Wilkins; 1985.
2. Shibasaki H, Kuriowa Y: Electroencephalographic correlates of myoclonus. *Electroencephalog Clin Neurolphysiol* 1975, 39:455–463.
3. Shibasaki H, Yamashita Y, Kuriowa Y: Electroencephalographic studies of myoclonus: myoclonus-related cortical spikes and high amplitude somatosensory evoked potentials. *Brain* 1978, 101:447–460.
4. Obeso JA, Artieda J, Burleigh AL: Clinical aspects of negative myoclonus. *Adv Neurol* 1995, 67:1–9.
5. Delgado-Escuota AV, Serratosa JM, Medina MT: Myoclonic Seizures and Progressive Myoclonic Epilepsy Syndromes. In *The Treatment of Epilepsy: Principles and Practice*, edn 2. Edited by Wyllie E. Baltimore: Williams & Wilkins; 1996: 467–483
6. Shibasaki H, Yamashita Y, Tobimatsu S, Neshige R: Electroencephalographic correlates of myoclonus. *Adv Neurol* 1986, 43:357–372.
7. Young RH, Shahani BT: Asterixis: one type of negative myoclonus. *Adv Neurol* 43:137–156.

MOVEMENT DISORDERS INDUCED BY DOPAMINE RECEPTOR BLOCKING AGENTS

- ◆ Tardive Dyskinesia Syndromes
- ◆ Oculogyric Crisis

Dopamine receptor blocking agents may cause a variety of acute, subacute, and chronic movement disorders. The acute disorders include acute dystonic reaction and acute akathisia. These tend to resolve spontaneously and upon discontinuation of the offending agent.

Tardive Dyskinesia Syndromes

The tardive dyskinesia syndromes are late-appearing involuntary movements resulting from chronic administration of dopamine receptor blocking agents. These syndromes present a range of movement disorder phenomenology, the best recognized of which is the classical orobuccolingual tardive dyskinesia, causing repetitive stereotyped chewing or lip pursing movements (Table 8-1, see Fig. 8-2).

In addition, other distinct tardive subsyndromes include tardive dystonia and tardive akathisia. Tardive dystonia is characterized by sustained torsional movements, often involving the cranial structures, neck, arms, and trunk, sometimes causing retrocollis and backwards trunk arching [1] (see Figs. 8-3 and 8-4). Tardive akathisia is late-occuring or persisting inner restlessness accompanied by external signs of restless behavior [2]. All late-appearing involuntary movements caused by dopamine receptor blocking agents may persist indefinitely despite discontinuation of the medication. Every patient treated with these agents should be informed of this possibility before starting therapy (Table 8-2).

Oculogyric Crisis

Oculogyric crisis is an acute dystonic reaction of the extra-ocular muscles, causing forced, sustained ocular deviation, usually upwards. The oculogyric crisis is often associated with retrocollis, forced jaw opening, and tongue protrusion. Patients may be able to force the eyes to mid-position, but the ocular deviation returns. At one time, oculogyric crises occurred

Table 8-1. Movement Disorders Induced by Dopamine-Receptor Blocking Agents

Movement disorders	Time course	Description	Treatment
Acute dystonic reaction	Immediate, acute; usually within first days of treatment, sometimes following first dose	Abnormal sustained muscle contractions or postures, most often affecting extraocular muscles (oculogyric crisis), neck, face, or trunk	Administer parenteral anticholinergics or antihistamines, remove offending neuroleptic
Acute akathisia	Acute, immediate	Acute state of inner restlessness	Self-limited upon discontinuation of neuroleptics
Neuroleptic-induced parkinsonism	Subacute, insidious	Dose-related parkinsonism, with rigidity, bradykinesia, postural instability, and all other clinical features of idiopathic Parkinson's disease	Reduce or withdraw neuroleptic, administer amantadine, or anticholinergics

Tardive syndromes

Abnormal involuntary movements caused by exposure to neuroleptic dopamine-receptor blocking agents, persisting for at least 1 month after withdrawal of the inciting drug

Classical tardive dyskinesia	Chronic, late, persistent	Repetitive, orobuccolingual chewing movements; tongue popping	Administer parenteral anticholinergics or antihistamines, remove offending neuroleptic
			Usually self-limited upon discontinuation of neuroleptics
			Reduce or withdraw neuroleptic, administer amantadine, or anticholinergics
Tardive dystonia		Sustained involuntary torsional movements of neck, trunk, oral region, or face	Administer reserpine, tetrabenazine, clozapine,

	Onset	Clinical features	Treatment
Tardive akathisia		Sensation of inner restlessness and intolerance of remaining still, with overt movements of restlessness, pacing, marching in place, fidgetiness	Administer anticholinergics, reserpine, or tetrabenazine Reserpine Tetrabenazine
Withdrawal-emergence syndrome	Occurs following abrupt withdrawal from chronic neuroleptic therapy; usually occurs in children	Generalized choreic movements involving trunk, limbs, neck, and rarely, face	Spontaneous resolution; movements resolve immmediately if neuroleptics are reinstated
Neuroleptic malignant syndrome	Begins abruptly while on neuroleptic or when stable dose of neuroleptic is suddenly reduced or discontinued	Fever, autonomic hyperactivity, muscle rigidity, and alteration of mental status	Discontinuation of neuroleptics; administer bromocriptine; dantrolene

exclusively in patients with encephalitis; afterwards, these individuals developed post-encephalitic parkinsonism and recurrent attacks of oculogyric crisis. At present, the commonest cause of oculogyric crisis is an acute dystonic reaction caused by a dopamine receptor blocking agent. The reaction usually occurs within 72 hours of beginning treatment, but may also occur following an abrupt escalation in neuroleptic dose in a chronically treated patient. The onset of an oculogyric crisis may be paroxysmal or stuttering. The attack is usually aborted with anticholinergic medication, such as benztropine 2 mg intravenously or intramuscularly, or diphenhydramine 50 mg intravenously or intramuscularly (Fig. 8-1).

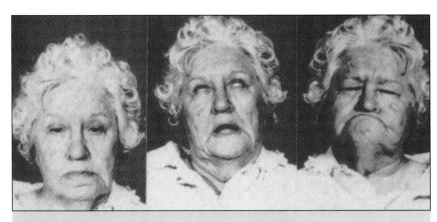

FIGURE 8-1 A patient experiencing an oculogyric crisis. (*From* Fitzgerald and colleague (3); with permission.)

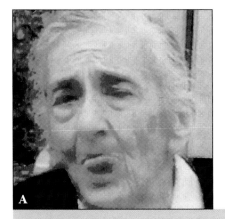
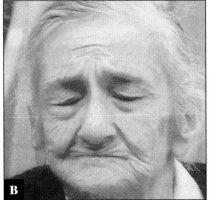

FIGURE 8-2 A patient with classic tardive dyskinesia of the oral-buccal-lingual type. **A**, Tongue popping movements. **B**, Other mouthing movements and eyelid closure.

Table 8-2. Drugs That May Cause Tardive Syndromes

Indication	Drug class	Drug name	Trade name
Antipsychotics	Phenothiazine	Chlorpromazine	Thorazine (SmithKline Beecham, Philadelphia, PA)
		Trifluopromazine	Vesprin (Apothecon, New York, NY)
		Thioridazine	Mellaril (Sandoz, East Hanover, NJ)
		Mesoridazine	Serentil (Boehringer Ingelheim, Ridgefield, CT)
		Trifluoperazine	Stelazine (SmithKline Beecham, Philadelphia, PA)
		Perphenazine	Trilafon (Schering, Kenilworth, NJ), Triavil (Merck, West Point, PA)
		Fluphenazine	Prolixin (Apothecon, New York, NY), Permitil (Schering, Kenilworth, NJ)
		Pimozide	Orap (Lemmon, Sellersville, PA)
		Acetophenazine	Tindal (Schering, Kenilworth, NJ)
	Thioxanthene	Chlorprothixene	Taractan (Hoffmann-LaRoche, Nutley, NJ)
		Thiothixene	Navane (Roerig, New York, NY)
	Butyrophenone	Haloperidol	Haldol (McNeil, Fort Washington, PA)
		Droperidol	Inapsine, Innovar (Janssen, Titusville, NJ)
	Dibenzepin	Loxapine	Loxitane (Lederle, Wayne, NJ), Doxolin (Miles, Elkhart, IN)
	Indolone	Molindone	Moban (Dupont Merck, Wilmington, DE), Lidone (Abbott, Abbott Park, IL)
	Pyrimidinone	Risperidone	Risperdal (Janssen, Titusville, NJ)
	Substituted benzamide	Tiapride	
		Sulpiride	
		Cleboride	
		Remoxipride	
Drugs used as anti-emetics, cough suppressants, or as treatment for intractable hiccoughs	Phenothiazine	Prochlorperazine	Compazine (SmithKline Beecham, Philadelphia, PA)
		Promethazine	Phenergan (Wyeth-Ayerst, Philadelphia, PA)
		Chlorpromazine	Thorazine (SmithKline Beecham, Philadelphia, PA)
		Triethylperazine	Torecan (Roxane Laboratories, Columbus, OH)
		Triflupromazine	Vesprin (Apothecon, New York, NY)
	Substituted benzamide	Metoclopramide	Reglan (A.H. Robins, Richmond, VA)
Antidepressant	Tricyclic	Amoxapine	Asendin (Lederle, Wayne, NJ)
Antihypertensive	Calcium channel blockers	Flunarizine	Triavil
		Cinnarizine	

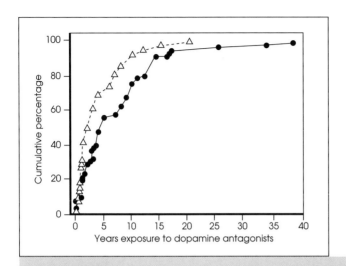

FIGURE 8-3 Relationship between exposure to neuroleptics and development of tardive dystonia. The cumulative percentage of patients with tardive dystonia is shown in relation to years of exposure to dopamine receptor antagonists in two different series of patients. The first series (*black circles*) comprises 67 patients followed at Columbia-Presbyterian Medical Center, and the second group (*open triangles*) consists of 43 patients reported in the literature before 1986. In both groups, cases of tardive dystonia developed shortly after exposure to neuroleptics, and no minimum safe duration of exposure was detected. (*Adapted from* Kang and colleague (1); with permission.)

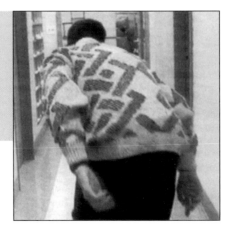

FIGURE 8-4 A patient with tardive dystonia showing flexion of his trunk as he walks. The elbows are extended and the wrists flexed. More common than trunk flexion in tardive dystonia is trunk extension with opisthotonus and retrocollis.

References

1. Kang UJ, Burke RE, Fahn S: Natural history and treatment of tardive dystonia. *Mov Disord* 1986, 1:193–208.
2. Burke RE, Kang UJ, Jankovic J, *et al.*: Tardive akathisia: an analysis of clinical features and response to open therapeutic trials. *Mov Disord* 1989, 4:157–175.
3. Fitzgerald PM, Jankovic J: Tardive oculogyric crises. *Neurology* 1989, 39:1434–1437.

Chapter 9

PERIPHERAL AND MISCELLANEOUS MOVEMENT DISORDERS

- ◆ Hemifacial Spasm

- ◆ Paroxysmal Disorders

- ◆ Psychogenic Movement Disorders

Hemifacial Spasm

Hemifacial spasm is a condition of recurrent unilateral contraction of the facial musculature innervated by CN VII. Hemifacial spasm was traditionally considered to be an idiopathic condition, but evidence from imaging studies and intra-operative visualization indicates that many, if not most, cases are associated with microvascular compression of the facial nerve. Rare causes of hemifacial spasm include posterior fossa tumors, aneurysms, arteriovenous malformations, arachnoid cysts, intrinsic glial tumors, brain stem infarction, and multiple sclerosis (Figs. 9-1 and 9-2) [1].

Surgical Treatment of Hemifacial Spasm

Hemifacial spasm can be effectively treated with injections of botulinum toxin or by decompression surgery. In a series of 782 microvascular decompression procedures for hemifacial spasm excellent results were achieved in 84%. Serious complications included ipsilateral deafness (2.6%), permanent facial paralysis (0.9%), brain stem infarction (0.3%), and death (0.1%) [1]. Microvascular decompression of the facial nerve is achieved by separating the vertebral artery from its point of contact with CN VII. A sponge, Teflon, or piece of muscle is interposed between the two structures (Figs. 9-3 and 9-4)

Paroxysmal Disorders

Paroxysmal disorders are conditions of recurrent episodes of sudden abnormal involuntary movements or ataxia. The attacks occur suddenly and without warning, but may be provoked by a variety of external factors. Episodes are not accompanied by loss of consciousness. Between attacks, patients are neurologically normal. Paroxysmal disorders may be hereditary, sporadic, or secondary to a structural defect (Tables 9-1 and 9-2).

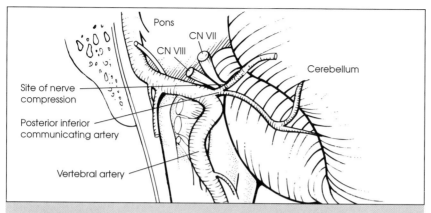

FIGURE 9-1 Compression of the facial nerve exit zone by the vertebral and posterior inferior cerebellar arteries in a patient with hemifacial spasm. (*Adapted from* Jannetta (2); with permission.)

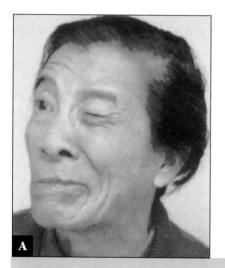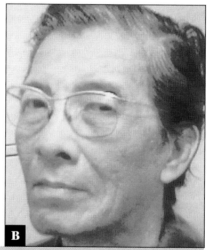

FIGURE 9-2 A patient with hemifacial spasm, before (**A**) and after (**B**) being treated with injections of botulinum toxin.

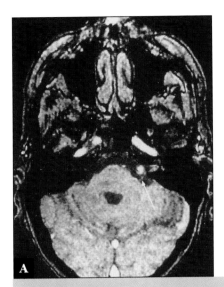

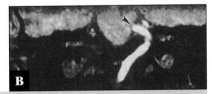

FIGURE 9-3 Magnetic resonance imaging (MRI) of a patient with a left hemifacial spasm. The MRI reveals an ectatic basilar artery contacting CN VII (**A**, *white arrow*; **B**, *black arrowhead*) in the left cerebellopontine angle. (*From* Adler and colleagues (3).)

FIGURE 9-4

Surgical treatment of hemifacial spasm: left retromastoid craniectomy (magnification x 16). *a.* Retractor on cerebellum; *b.* CN IX (hypoglossal nerve) and X (vagus nerve); *c.* vertebral artery; *d.* CN VIII (vestibulocochlear nerve); *e.* CN VII (facial nerve); and *f.* sponge prosthesis in place. (*From* Jannetta and colleagues (4); with permission.)

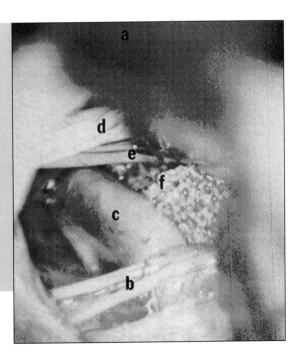

Table 9-1. Paroxysmal Ataxias

Type	Age at onset, y	Clinical features	Precipitants	Frequency	Duration of attacks	Treatment	Genetic linkage
Neuromyotonia-myokymia	2–15	Weakness, ataxia, dysarthria, tremor, facial twitching	Startle, movement, exercise, fatigue, excitement	Up to 15 per day	Usually 2–10 minutes	Anticonvulsants	12p13 K+ channel
Vestibular	Usually 5–15	Ataxia, vertigo, nystagmus, dysarthria, headache, ptosis, ocular palsy, cerebellar atrophy	Stress, alcohol, fatigue, exercise, caffeine	Daily to every 2 months	Usually hours	Acetazolamide	19p

The paroxysmal ataxias are a clinically heterogeneous group of disorders that is in the process of re-classification according to genetic linkage data. Like the periodic paralysis syndromes, startle disease, and other paroxysmal disorders, it is possible that the paroxysmal ataxias are caused by an ion channel mutation. (Adapted from Browne and colleagues [5]; with permission; and Vahedi and colleagues [6]; with permission.)

Table 9-2. Paroxysmal Choreoathetosis

	Inheritance	Male to female ratio	Age at onset, y	Frequency	Attack duration	Precipitant	Treatment	Genetic linkage
Paroxysmal kinesigenic choreoathetosis (PKC)	AD	4:1	1–40	100 daily to 1 monthly	< 5 minutes	Sudden movement, startle, hyper-ventilation	Anticonvulsants, acetazolamide, antimuscarinics	2p 31-36[9]
Paroxysmal nonkinesigenic dystonia choreo-athetosis (PDC)	AD	1.4:1	1–30	3 daily to 2 yearly	2 minutes–4 hours	Occurs at rest, caffeine, alcohol	Clonazepam, benzodi-azepines	

The paroxysmal dyskinesias are a heterogeneous group of disorders initially classified on the basis of clinical criteria. Increasingly, genetics linkage studies will enable a re-classification of these disorders based on genetic defects. Several families have been described that have unique phenotypes, such as paroxysmal choreoathetosis and spasticity, mapped to a potassium channel gene on chromosome 1p [10]. AD—Autosomal dominant. (Adapted from Mount and colleague [7] and Lance [8]).

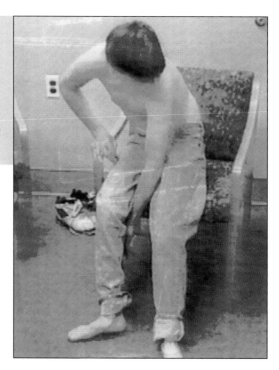

FIGURE 9-5

A patient with paroxysmal kinesigenic dyskinesia, causing involuntary neck rotation and right arm posturing, induced by sudden movement and lasting only a few seconds.

Psychogenic Movement Disorders

Psychogenic movement disorders are abnormal movements that do not result from a known organic cause but are caused by psychologic conditions. Most psychogenic movements can be placed into a specific category of abnormal movement such as tremor, chorea, dystonia, myoclonus, parkinsonism, or gait disturbance. Psychogenic movements that are generalized may overlap with the symptomatology of epilepsy. The two most important clues suggesting a possible psychogenic cause are abnormal movements that are incongruous with typical organic disease, and movements that are inconsistent or fluctuate during the examination. The importance of an accurate diagnosis cannot be overstated, and there is no substitute for a careful assessment by an experienced observer of movement disorders. The diagnosis is certain only when the movement disorder is persistently relieved by psychotherapy. The psychiatric diagnoses in cases of psychogenic movement disorders include conversion disorder, somatization disorder, factitious disorder, and malingering. Effective treatment generally requires a combination of intensive psychotherapy, physical therapy, pharmacotherapy, and other rehabilitation techniques (Table 9-3 and Fig. 9-5).

Table 9-3. Psychogenic Movement Disorders

Clinical features of psychogenic movement disorders

Abrupt onset, with clear inciting event

Multiple movement disorder manifestations

Variable and inconsistent motor manifestations, fluctuating within the same examination session

Motor manifestations that are incongruous with organic pathology

Movements increase or become more elaborate when examination focuses upon the affected body part

Movements diminish or resolve when not the clear focus of attention or inquiry

Movements diminish or resolve during tests requiring concentration or other tasks

Hyperekplexia, or excessive startle response

Movements respond to placebo or suggestion

Associated false or incongruous neurologic signs

Associated psychiatric features

Movement disorder resolves with psychotherapy, or when patient is unaware of being observed

Additional features of psychogenic tremor

Tremor similar in all positions and at rest, posture-holding, and with action

Variability of examination: changes in frequency, distribution, direction, and amplitude

Spontaneous remission

Selective or intermittent disability

Entrainment of tremor by tests of coordination

Additional features of psychogenic dystonia

Onset of dystonia at rest

Onset in foot in adults

Specific incongruities: absence of dystonic tremor, absence of null point, absence of modifying sensory tricks

Spontaneous pain with passive movement

Startle-induced elaboration of dystonic postures

Abrupt changes in dystonia

Contractures do not exclude diagnosis

(From Williams and colleagues [11]; with permission.)

References

1. Barker FG, Jannetta PJ, Bissonette DJ, *et al.*: Microvascular decompression for hemifacial spasm. *J Neurosurg* 1995, 82:201–210.

2. Jannetta PJ: Cranial Rhizotomies. In *Neurological Surgery*, vol. 6, edn 3. Edited by Youmans JR. Philadelphia: WB Saunders; 1990.

3. Adler CH, Zimmerman RA, Savino PJ, *et al.*: Hemifacial spasm: evaluation by MRI and MR tomographic angiography. *Ann Neurol* 1992, 32:502–506.

4. Jannetta PJ, Abbasy M, Maroon JC, *et al.*: Etiology and definitive microsurgical treatment of hemifacial spasm. *J Neurosurg* 1977, 47:321–328.

5. Browne DL, Gaucher ST, Nutt TG, *et al.*: Episodic ataxia/myokymia syndrome is associated with point mutations in the human potassium channel gene KCNAI. *Nat Genet* 1994, 8:136–140.

6. Vahedi K, Joutel A, van Bogaert P, *et al.*: A gene for hereditary cerebellar ataxia maps to chromosome 19p. *Ann Neurol* 1995, 37:289–293.

7. Mount LA, Reback S: Familial paroxysmal choreoathetosis. *Arch Neurol Psychiatr* 1940, 44:841–847.

8. Lance JW: Familial paroxysmal dystonic choreoathetosis and its differentiation from related syndrome. *Ann Neurol* 1977, 2:285–293.

9. Fink JH, Hedera P, Mathay JG, Albin RL; Paroxysmal dystonic choreoathetosis linked to chromosome 2q. Clinical analysis and proposed pathophysiology. *Neurology* 1997, 49:177–183.

10. Auberger G, Razlaff T, Lunkes A, *et al.*: A gene for autosomal dominant paroxysmal choreoathetosis/spasticiy (CSE) maps to the vicinity of a potassium channel gene cluster on chromosome 1p. *Geneomics* 1996, 31:90–94.

11. Williams DT, Ford B, Fahn S: Phenomenology and psychopathology related to psychogenic movement disorders. *Adv Neurol* 65:231–257.

Chapter 10

AGENTS FOR TREATING MOVEMENT DISORDERS

- ◆ Basal Ganglia

- ◆ Dopamine Synthesis and Metabolism

- ◆ Treatment Approach to Parkinson's Disease

- ◆ Treatment Approach to Hyperkinetic Movement Disorders

- ◆ Drugs Used in the Treatment of Movement Disorders

The clinical approach to treating movement disorders emphasizes symptomatic pharmacologic therapy. Many medications are available for the treatment of Parkinson's disease and other movement disorders, many of which have a specific target or site of action within the central nervous system (CNS). Knowledge of the relevant neuroanatomy and biochemistry is important for those using the medications discussed here.

Basal Ganglia

Although the specific pathologic and biochemical basis for many movement disorders is not known, the clinical manifestations often implicate the basal ganglia as the primary site of disturbance. The basal ganglia are a group of interconnected subcortical nuclei, including the caudate, globus pallidus, putamen, subthalamic nucleus, and substantia nigra (see Fig.1-1 on page 5) [1]. Normal function of these structures and their connections is required for normal motor control and posture. The basal ganglia exert an inhibitory influence on the premotor area of the cerebral cortex by way of output from the ventrolateral thalamus. The thalamus receives projections from the globus pallidus and substantia nigra reticulata, which in turn receive projections from the striatum, an important nuclear group comprising the caudate and putamen. A major afferent projection to the striatum is the nigrostriatal dopaminergic pathway, which originates in the substantia nigra and terminates in the striatum [2]. Degeneration of the nigrostriatal pathway in Parkinson's disease is responsible for the cardinal features of the condition, including the tremor at rest, rigidity, and bradykinesia. Diminished dopaminergic input to the striatum is believed to result in decreased thalamocortical excitation of the premotor region. Hemiballism, characterized by irregular flailing and writhing movements of the limbs on one side of the body, results from a lesion of the contralateral subthalamic nucleus, leading to excessive excitatory drive of the cortex by the thalamus. Chorea is character-

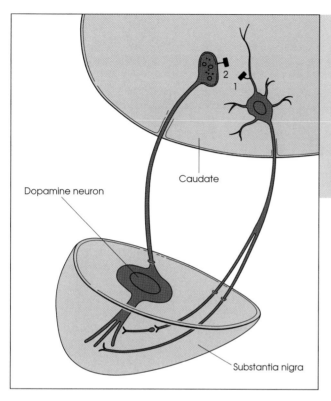

FIGURE 10-1 A dopaminergic neuron of the striatonigral pathway, with its cell body in the substantia nigra (pars compacta) and its terminal dendrites in the caudate nucleus. The neuron releases dopamine from its presynaptic membrane (3) into the synaptic cleft, where it acts on the dopamine receptor of a striatal neuron (2). (*From* Cooper and colleagues (3); with permission.)

Caudate

Dopamine neuron

Substantia nigra

ized by irregular, random, jerky movements that originate from a lesion of the caudate nucleus. The putamen is more commonly involved in dystonia, a condition of sustained twisting movements and postures.

In Parkinson's disease, the major class of pharmacologic agents is dopaminergic drugs, which act on the nigrostriatal pathway. Conceptually the cell body of a striatonigral neuron is in the substantia nigra pars compacta, and its terminal dendrites synapse in the striatum (Fig. 10-1) [3]. The nigrostriatal neuron synthesizes dopamine and stores the neurotransmitter in presynaptic vesicles. When dopamine is released into the synaptic cleft, the neurotransmitter diffuses to the postsynaptic membrane and interacts with specific striatal dopamine receptors, designated D_1 and D_2. The striatum also contains a high level of cholinergic markers, although the precise role of cholinergic systems in normal motor control is uncertain. Anticholinergic drugs play an important role in the treatment of Parkinson disease and dystonia.

Dopamine Synthesis and Metabolism

In the mammalian brain, the highest levels of dopamine are found in the striatum. The first step in dopamine biosynthesis is the uptake from the bloodstream of amino acid L-tyrosine. Tyrosine is converted to 3,4-dihydroxyphenylalanine (L-DOPA) by the enzyme tyrosine hydroxylase, which is the rate-limiting step of the pathway. The final step in dopamine biosynthesis is the conversion of L-DOPA to dopamine by the enzyme dopa decarboxylase. Dopamine accumulates within storage granules of presynaptic nerve terminals and is released during nerve stimulation. The action of dopamine is terminated primarily by reuptake of the neurotransmitter by the presynaptic neuron. The metabolic degradation of dopamine is performed chiefly by two enzymes, monoamine oxidase (MAO) and catechol-O-methyltransferase (COMT). MAO is present in the human brain in two types, A and B, distinguished by substrate specificity and sensitivity to various enzyme inhibitors [3]. Selegiline is a selective inhibitor of the MAO-B type. Figure 10-2 illustrates a CNS dopaminergic neuron, with the life cycle of dopamine and the steps at which pharmacologic intervention may occur.

Treatment Approach to Parkinson's Disease

The cardinal symptoms of Parkinson's disease are rigidity, bradykinesia, postural impairment, and tremor at rest, all of which relate to a disturbance in the function of the nigrostriatal dopaminergic pathway. A parkinsonian syndrome may result from presynaptic degeneration of the pathway, postsynaptic receptor alternations or degeneration, medications that block dopamine receptors, agents that disrupt the metabolism of dopamine, specific nigrostriatal toxins, and other conditions. Symptoms of Parkinson's disease have been conceptualized as an imbalance between striatal cholinergic and dopaminergic influences on motor function. Viewed according to this pharmacologic model, treatment of parkinsonism may consist of increasing dopaminergic drive by supplying levodopa or other agonists or by reducing cholinergic drive with anticholinergic medications. Pharmacologic strategies to enhance dopaminergic function include attempts to increase the synthesis of dopamine (levodopa), increase release of presynaptic dopamine (amantadine), decrease dopamine synaptic reuptake, stimulate postsynaptic dopamine receptors (bromocriptine, pergolide, pramipexole, and ropinerole), or inhibit metabolic enzymes (selegiline or the COMT inhibitors, entacapone and tolcapone). Dopaminergic and anticholinergic medications remain the primary categories of pharmacologic treatment for Parkinson's disease and related disorders. Levodopa is the pro-

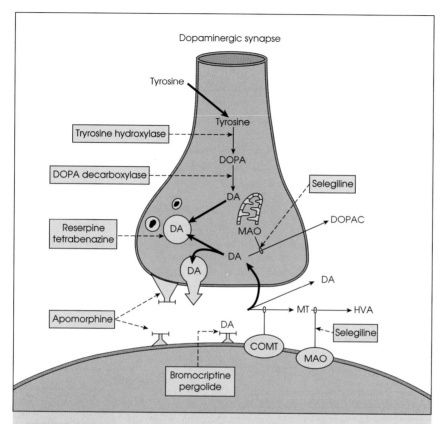

FIGURE 10-2 Schematic model of a central doapminergic neuron indicating the synthetic pathway for dopamine, dopamine metabolism, and sites of action of different drugs. COMT—catechol-O-methyltransferase; DA—dopamine; DOPAC—dihydroxyphenlyacetic acid; HVA—homovanillic acid; MAO—monoamine oxidase; MT—methoxytryptamine. (*From* Cooper and colleagues (2); with permission.)

totype dopaminergic agent, and trihexyphenidyl is the prototype centrally acting anticholinergic drug. The six currently available dopaminergic drugs in the United States are amantadine, bromocriptine, pergolide, pramipexole, ropinerole, and levodopa.

The management of Parkinson's disease is symptomatic for the most part. Pharmacotherapy is directed at suppressing symptoms, and the specific choice of therapy depends on the severity of the symptom, the degree of overall disability, the tolerance of adverse effects, and the presence of complications. Important nonpharmacologic interventions include exercise, nutrition, education, and support. Mild Parkinson's disease that is charac-

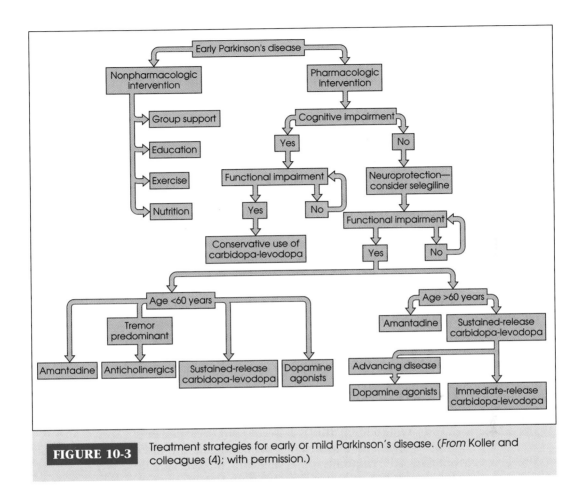

FIGURE 10-3   Treatment strategies for early or mild Parkinson's disease. (*From* Koller and colleagues (4); with permission.)

terized by a tremor at rest often is treated initially with amantadine or anticholinergic agents. Neuroprotective treatment in the form of selegiline is often used as an initial therapy in early Parkinson's disease, although the current role of this agent in modern clinical practice is not clear. For functional difficulty, dopaminergic medication is prescribed. The relative importance of levodopa and the dopamine agonists is uncertain. At one time, the dopamine agonists were used in patients already taking levodopa, and who were experiencing levodopa-induced motor fluctuations. Now, dopamine agonists often are used before levodopa. Levodopa remains the most potent symptomatic antiparkinsonian agent. How levodopa influences the long-term course of Parkinson's disease is unknown, but many neurologists reserve this drug for later stages of the disease. Figure 10-3 shows approaches to management of early Parkinson's disease. Additional problems arising as complications of Parkinson's disease often may be treated with specific therapy following appropriate evaluation.

Insomnia, depression, constipation, urinary urgency, hypersalivation, leg cramps, orthostatic hypotension, and other problems may all be treated in conjunction with the parkinsonian symptoms. A complete discussion is beyond the scope of this chapter. Tricyclic antidepressants are useful in depression and insomnia and may reduce hypersalivation. Cisapride is helpful in treating gastric reflux in Parkinson's disease patients.

Physicians who care for patients with Parkinson's disease are aware that treatment is more often limited not by inadequate therapeutic response but by dose-limiting side effects. Many patients with Parkinson's disease are elderly, with enhanced susceptibility to adverse drug effects. Because Parkinson's disease is a chronic, progressive disorder, the physician must continually optimize medical therapy. Although pharmacotherapy for Parkinson's disease is often extremely efficacious, it is not advisable to eradicate every symptom of the disease by aggressive dosing because this approach increases the risk of adverse effects. In general, it is prudent to establish a specific therapeutic goal whenever a pharmacologic change is made. Whether the goal is reduction of a parkinsonian symptom or allevi-ation of an adverse medication effect, the change in therapy should have a defined purpose. Avoiding or limiting adverse effects is critically important because a side effect may lead to the incorrect conclusion that a drug is harmful and should be stopped. Knowledge of the adverse effects of each medication used for Parkinson's disease is required for proper management.

Managing Complications of Levodopa Therapy

Most patients with early, typical idiopathic Parkinson's disease experience a beneficial response to levodopa replacement treatment. In the most favorable circumstances, all symptoms of Parkinson's disease can be eliminated, allowing the patient complete freedom from tremor, rigidity, or bradykinesia. With time, as the degeneration of the nigrostriatal dopaminergic system continues, the effectiveness of levodopa therapy diminishes, and various complications supervene. These complications may include loss of response to the medication, shortened duration of beneficial effect, wearing-off fluctuations, drug-induced dyskinesias, and toxic adverse effects of the medication (Fig. 10-4) [7].

Fluctuations

The wearing-off phenomenon is the return of parkinsonism that occurs as the peripheral levels of levodopa decline after an oral dose. Wearing-off fluctuations may be gradual, sudden, predictable, or unpredictable. The problem may be remedied initially by attempts to shorten the levodopa dosage interval, by prolonging or potentiating the effect of levodopa, or by adding other antiparkinson agents. Mild wearing off can be helped by

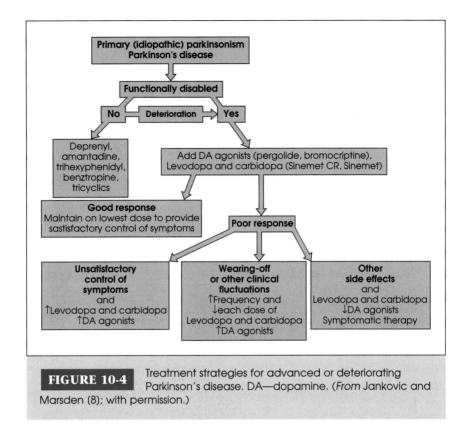

FIGURE 10-4 Treatment strategies for advanced or deteriorating Parkinson's disease. DA—dopamine. (*From* Jankovic and Marsden (8); with permission.)

adding deprenyl, which may act by prolonging the effect of levodopa. Substituting the regular preparation of levodopa with the long-acting (controlled-release) levodopa-carbidopa preparation (Sinemet CR) also may be beneficial. Sudden or unpredictable wearing off can be treated by the ingestion of a crushed or dissolved levodopa-carbidopa tablet, which can be absorbed rapidly on an empty stomach, so that the effect takes place within 15 minutes in a patient who normally responds to the medication. Apomorphine subcutaneous injections can quickly treat wearing-off fluctuations, although the drug induces nausea, necessitating pretreatment with domperidone.

Local gastric and dietary factors may contribute to wearing off and unresponsiveness to levodopa. Delayed gastric emptying may impair the transit to the small intestine, where levodopa is absorbed. Dietary protein interferes with both the absorption of levodopa from the gut and the passage of levodopa across the blood–brain barrier. The amino acids resulting from protein breakdown in the gut compete with levodopa for a nonspecific carrier to obtain access to the CNS. Therefore, patients with disabling wearing-off fluctuations often need to take levodopa well before meals, and they must often limit protein intake during the day to optimize levodopa effectiveness. Other measures have been reported for patients with severe, disabling wearing-off fluctuations that are not correctable by simple pharmacologic changes. These include use of liquid levodopa [9], continuous infusion of levodopa via a duodenal catheter [10], and adjuvant medications, such as COMT inhibitors [11], that inhibit the peripheral metabolism of levodopa.

Dyskinesias

Levodopa can induce involuntary choreic movements that are dose related. The movements, when mild and nondisabling, indicate slight levodopa toxicity. Severe generalized choreiform dyskinesias are more likely to occur in patients with advanced Parkinson's disease who require increasing doses of levodopa to control parkinsonism. The simplest treatment for levodopa-induced dyskinesias is to lower the dose or decrease the bioavailability of levodopa. Patients with moderate or severe Parkinson's disease, however, may not tolerate dose reduction. Moreover, some people with Parkinson's disease experience alternating severe wearing-off fluctuations and violent levodopa-induced dyskinesias, with little or no normal motor function. Therapeutic approaches to this problem include the administration of small, more frequent doses of levodopa, aiming for a more uniform plasma level of the drug. Use of the long-acting preparation and concomitant administration of agonists may help. Other techniques for controlling severe dyskinesias include the administration of clozapine [12] as well as continuous infusions of liquid levodopa [13].

Anticholinergics

Use and Indications

The basal ganglia contain a high level of cholinergic neuronal markers. In Parkinson's disease, selective degeneration of striatonigral neurons allows a putative overactivity of cholinergic output. Historically, anticholinergic medication for Parkinson's disease preceded the advent of dopaminergic therapy. Numerous anticholinergic medications are available, each with similar mechanisms of action, therapeutic effects, and adverse effects (Table 10-1). The class of agents consists of centrally acting muscarinic acetylcholine receptor antagonists, epitomized by trihexiphenidyl. In Parkinson's disease, anticholinergic drugs can reduce tremor. Other cardinal symptoms of Parkinson's disease, such as rigidity, bradykinesia, and postural instability, however, generally resist anticholinergic therapy. These medications are often a first-line treatment for patients with mild Parkinson's disease who manifest primarily a unilateral rest tremor. Anti-

Table 10-1. The Equivalent Doses of Anticholinergics

Benztropine (Cogentin, Merck, West Point, PA) 1 mg

Biperiden (Akineton, Knoll, Mount Olive, NJ) 2 mg

Trihexyphenidyl (Artane, Lederle, Philadelphia, PA) 2 mg

Procyclidine (Kemadrin, Glaxo Wellcome, Research Triangle Park, NC) 5 mg

Orphenadrine (Disipal, 3M Pharmaceuticals, St. Paul, MN) 25 mg

Ethopropazine (Parsidol, Parke-Davis, Morris Plains, NJ) 50 mg

Diphenhydramine (Benadryl, Parke-Davis, Morris Plains, NJ) 100 mg

(Adapted from Cedarbaum and colleague [6]; with permission.)

cholinergics also inhibit salivary gland secretion, and these drugs may help the drooling associated with Parkinson's disease.

Potential Adverse Effects

Anticholinergic agents can produce reversible, dose-dependent muscarinic side effects. Constipation, urinary retention, dry mouth, papillary dilatation (mydriasis), paralysis of accommodation (cycloplegia), and confusion may result. Confusion seems especially likely in the elderly patient, and many Parkinson's disease patients cannot tolerate anticholinergic medication. Often, adverse effects can be avoided or limited by providing low starting doses and increasing by small increments. As a rule, we do not recommend using anticholinergics in patients older than 70 years. Tolerance may develop to both the therapeutic effect of the medication and the adverse effects. Each anticholinergic agent may have slight chemical differences, accounting for minute variations in tolerance between patients. In patients receiving an anticholinergic medication for Parkinson's disease or dystonia, sudden cessation of the drug may induce a rebound in symptoms.

Treatment Approach to Hyperkinetic Movement Disorders

Tourette Syndrome and Related Tic Disorders

Tics are involuntary, rapid, brief, purposeless, repetitive, and stereotyped movements that compose the core symptoms of Tourette syndrome and related tic disorders (see Chapter 5). Tics may consist of simple or complex motor or vocal manifestations. Tic disorders are conditions of recurrent tics, classified by clinical manifestations, symptom duration, and age at onset. The precise neuroanatomic and biochemical substrates of tic disorders are not known, but experimental work and the responses to various pharmacologic agents implicate abnormal neurotransmitter functioning. A disturbance in dopaminergic transmission is supported by the suppression of tics that can be achieved by dopamine receptor–blocking agents, such as haloperidol, or dopamine-depleting agents, such as reserpine or tetrabenazine. Benzodiazepines, which enhance the effect of the inhibitory neurotransmitter γ-aminobutyric acid (GABA), also are effective in tic suppression.

The first-line agents for the treatment of tic disorders are clonazepam and clonidine. More potent medications include the catecholamine-depleting agents reserpine and tetrabenazine, although these medications are restricted by the development of side effects and by limited market availability. The neuroleptics haloperidol, pimozide, and risperidone are potent suppressors of tics, but long-term administration of these drugs carries the risk of development of additional involuntary movements, such as tardive dyskinesias and dystonia. Clonazepam is also useful in the treatment of epilepsy, myoclonus, and anxiety.

Dystonia

Dystonia is the term for involuntary, torsional movements that can lead to characteristic postures and deformities (see Chapter 3). Dystonic movements can be rapid or slow, brief or prolonged, random, irregular, or tremulous, but the defining feature of the movement is the twisting aspect, slightly sustained at the peak of contraction. Dystonia can be the unitary symptom of a disease, as in classic idiopathic torsion dystonia, or an accompaniment of other neurologic symptoms, including developmental delay, parkinsonism, spasticity, cognitive deficits, and other movement disorders. Dystonia is classified by anatomic distribution, age at onset, and etiology. Identification of the cause of dystonia is an important prelude to the choice of therapy. In general, dystonia restricted to a body part, such as focal brachial dystonia (writer's cramp) or cervical dystonia (torticollis), is best treated with localized injections of botulinum toxin. Widespread or generalized dystonia requires treatment with medication (Table 10-2).

Because dystonia is a rare condition, randomized, controlled, double-blind studies are few, and much of the therapeutic approach is based on small, open-label trials conducted at specialized centers for dystonia [14].

The precise neurochemical cause of dystonia is unknown, and treatment regimens have evolved on an empiric basis. Idiopathic childhood-onset dystonia, the classically described dystonia musculorum deformans, responds best to high doses of anticholinergics [5] (*eg*, trihexiphenidyl) and baclofen, often in combination. In dystonia, the therapeutic response may require doses greatly exceeding the standard guidelines listed in the *Physician's Desk Reference*. It is advisable to increase the dosage only in small increments to avoid or reduce the development of side effects. Mixed therapeutic success has been reported with other agents, including levodopa, clonazepam and other benzodiazepines, carbamazepine, haloperidol and other dopamine receptor–blocking drugs, and catecholamine depletors. Patients with generalized dystonia of childhood onset should always undergo a trial of levodopa because a small proportion have dopa-responsive dystonia, which is exquisitely sensitive to that medication. Tardive dystonia, induced by chronic exposure to neuroleptics, differs in its therapeutic response from idiopathic dystonia. Anticholinergic agents and catecholamine-depleting agents, such as reserpine and tetrabenazine, are most effective for this type of dystonia [15]. Dystonia resulting from anoxic and ischemic brain injury, metabolic disease, trauma, Wilson's disease, and other causes is treated symptomatically using combinations of the medications just listed. Acute dystonic reactions induced by neuroleptic administration are treated with anticholinergic medication, such as diphenhydramine (see Table 10-2).

Tremors

Tremors are rhythmical oscillations of a body part characterized by the alternating or simultaneous activation of agonist and antagonist muscles (see Chapter 6). Tremors are classified by distribution, clinical characteristics, frequency, or etiology. A useful clinical approach to diagnosing tremor is the determination of whether the tremor is present at rest, when holding a posture, or with various activities. A common condition treated by neurologists is essential tremor, a chronic tremor usually involving the arms and hands bilaterally, present with posture-holding and most tasks involving the hands, such as using eating utensils or writing. The condition is often familial and responsive to alcohol. Essential tremor is often termed a benign tremor because it is not a degenerative condition. Because essential tremor can interfere progressively with the performance of all tasks involving hand coordination, the condition may not necessarily seem benign. The decision to treat essential tremor is usually based on the degree of impairment caused by the tremor or the social embarrassment attended by its appearance. Several drugs are effective for essential tremor, including β-blockers such as propranolol and primidone (Table 10-3).

These drugs have other applications within neurology, and detailed descriptions of their pharmacology and side effects are found elsewhere in this book. When one agent does not produce a satisfactory result, a combination of medications, such as propranolol and mysoline together, may be helpful.

Table 10-2. Drug Treatment for Dystonia

Idiopathic dystonia

Generalized dystonia

    Anticholinergics

    Baclofen

    Clonazepam, diazepam, lorazepam

    Carbamazepine

    Dopamine-depleting and dopamine receptor-blocking agents: reserpine, tetrabenazine, haloperidol

Focal dystonia

    Botulinum toxin A

    Botulinum toxin B

    Anticholinergics

    Baclofen

Dopa-responsive dystonia

    Levodopa (low-dose)

Tardive dystonia

    Remove offending neuroleptic(s)

    Anticholinergics

    Dopamine-depleting agents: reserpine, tetrabenazine

    Clozapine (?)

Other symptomatic dystonia

    Baclofen

    Anticholinergics

    Clonazepam, diazepam, lorazepam

    Intrathecal baclofen

Table 10-3. Treatment of Tremors

Medication	Usual daily dose range	Potential side effects
Propranolol	80–240 mg/d, in 2 or 3 divided doses	Fatigue, sedation, depression, hypotension, bradycardia, impotence
Metoprolol	100–200 mg/d, in 2 or 3 divided doses	Same as propranolol
Primidone	usually <250 mg/d	Sedation, confusion, ataxia, nausea

Myoclonus

Myoclonus is a brief, sudden, singular, shock-like muscle jerk (see Chapter 7). Recurrent or severe myoclonic jerking is characterized by its distribution over the body, its electrophysiologic characteristics, and its cause. The causes of pathologic myoclonus are numerous and include virtually every known type of brain or spinal cord lesion, whether metabolic, nutritional, degenerative, traumatic, vascular, infectious, hereditary, or toxic. Myoclonus can be a defining feature of many other medical and neurologic diseases. It can be associated with many other symptoms, including epilepsy (which can resemble myoclonus), dementia, growth retardation, poor coordination, visual disturbances, and others. The most useful medications for myoclonus are anticonvulsants, and two first-line drugs for myoclonus are clonazepam and valproic acid.

Wilson's Disease

Wilson's disease (hepatolenticular degeneration) results from a rare, autosomal recessive inborn error of copper metabolism [16] (see Chapter 3). The metabolic defect leads to the accumulation of copper in the body, which is deposited in several organs, causing widespread damage. Neurologic symptoms of Wilson's disease relate primarily to copper deposition in the basal ganglia. In the liver, copper deposition causes fatty infiltration, inflammation, and hepatocellular damage, leading to cirrhosis. Copper deposition in the kidney causes tubular and glomerular dysfunction. In the cornea, copper deposition in the Descemet membrane produces the pathognomonic brownish iris pigmentation, the Kayser-Fleischer ring, readily visible to inspection or slit-lamp examination. In the individual with sporadic or unsuspected Wilson's disease, the most common presenting symptoms are neurologic or psychiatric manifestations or symptoms and signs of liver disease. Although Wilson's disease is rare, the condition should never be overlooked because treatment in the early stages may reverse all symptoms and prevent further complications.

DRUGS USED IN THE TREATMENT OF MOVEMENT DISORDERS

Amantadine Hydrochloride
(Symmetrel)

Amantadine originally was used as a treatment for influenza A virus. Its effect on Parkinson's disease was noted fortuitously when patients with Parkinson's disease receiving this drug for the flu showed an amelioration of the parkinsonism. The mechanism of action of amantadine in Parkinson's disease is unknown, but the agent is believed to release dopamine from nerve terminals, making the neurotransmitter more available to activate postsynaptic dopaminergic receptors. Amantadine is not a direct anticholinergic but may induce side effects typical of anticholinergic agents.

Special Precautions

The dose of amantadine may need careful adjustment in patients with heart failure, renal disease, peripheral edema, or orthostatic hypotension.

Care should be exercised when administering this drug to patients with liver disease, recurrent eczematoid rash, dementia, or psychosis.

Patients taking amantadine who note blurred vision, sedation, or other central nervous system effects should be cautioned against driving or working in a setting that demands vigilance.

The safety of amantadine in pregnancy has not been established.

Amantadine should not be discontinued abruptly in a patient with advanced Parkinson's disease because this may precipitate a severe worsening of the condition. The dosage should be reduced gradually because rare cases of a neuroleptic malignant syndrome–like condition have followed sudden cessation of the drug.

If atropine-like side effects develop in a patient concurrently taking anticholinergic medications, the dosage of either amantadine or the anticholinergics may require reduction.

Dosage

Initial recommended dose is 100 mg/d. This can be increased to 100 mg twice a day within a week, if needed. Amantadine 100 mg four times daily is considered the upper dose and may benefit patients who are not treated adequately with lower doses or whose benefit from lower doses waned.

IN BRIEF

Indications

Monotherapy in early or mild Parkinson's disease; adjuvant agent in patients who take dopamine agonists, including levodopa; relief of tremor and bradykinesia in Parkinson's disease patients; neuroleptic-induced parkinsonism

Adverse Effects

Orthostatic hypotension, congestive heart failure, ankle edema, livedo reticularis, depression, hallucinations or psychosis, vivid dreams, nausea, diarrhea, dizziness, insomnia or somnolence, nervousness, headache, dry mouth, constipation, urinary retention

Pharmacokinetics and Pharmacodynamics

Peak action: 4 h
Plasma half-life: 15–24 h

Prolonged Use

Many patients taking amantadine may lose their responsiveness to the drug after several months, but a minority derive benefit for years.

Availability

Capsules—100 mg   Syrup—50 mg/5 mL

Apomorphine

Apomorphine is a direct-acting dopamine agonist with affinity for D_1 and D_2 receptors. The principal advantage of this dopamine agonist when given subcutaneously is its rapid onset of action. Therefore, the drug is useful in the treatment of Parkinson's disease patients with rapid or unpredictable off-fluctuations of increased parkinsonism [17]. The antiparkinsonian effect of apomorphine is not superior to that of levodopa, and the effectiveness of levodopa in relieving Parkinson's disease symptoms can predict the response of apomorphine.

Patients receiving apomorphine injections should be treated with domperidone to prevent the nausea and emesis that apomorphine can induce.

Dosage

Testing of apomorphine is most safely accomplished in a hospital or other carefully monitored setting. A test dose of apomorphine should be given during an off-fluctuation, when the patient is experiencing an increase in parkinsonian symptoms. An off period often can be provoked by withholding dopaminergic medication overnight. Beginning with a subcutaneous injection of apomorphine 0.5 or 1.0 mg, the dose may be repeated at 20-minute intervals until a beneficial response is seen. Most patients can expect to achieve a motor response equal to the optimal effect of levodopa by the time a cumulative apomorphine dose of 5 to 10 mg is reached. The lowest dose that provides an antiparkinsonian effect is the threshold dose. Once the threshold dose for responding to apomorphine has been determined, patients should inject themselves with approximately twice that amount subcutaneously at the beginning of an off-fluctuation. At the start of apomorphine therapy, determinations of upright and sitting blood pressure are required for 1 hour after a full clinical response. Injections can be given using a pen-shaped injecting device that can be prefilled with apomorphine and preset to deliver a specific amount of drug each time. Injections can be given subcutaneously into the abdominal wall although the thigh or proximal arm are also acceptable.

IN BRIEF

Indications

Off-fluctuations of increased parkinsonism

Adverse Effects

Nausea, vomiting, sedation, confusion, hallucinations, postural hypotension, dyskinesias, bleeding and infection at the site of repeated injections

Pharmacokinetics and Pharmacodynamics

Duration of action: 30–70 min
Onset of action: 5–15 min
Plasma half-life: 30 min

Patient Information

Patients planning to deliver self-injections must be trained in all aspects of dose adjustment and use of the injection device. Apomorphine is typically required during a period of increased parkinsonism when self-injection may be difficult or impractical, so the injection may require a care-giver. Patients who do not improve control over parkinsonian motor fluctuations despite improvement after single injections of apomorphine may be suitable candidates for a continuous subcutaneous apomorphine infusion, delivered by a portable pump system.

Bromocriptine
(Parlodel)

Bromocriptine is an ergot derivative that acts as a dopamine agonist at D_2 receptors, with mild antagonist activity at D_1 receptors. The drug also possesses weak α-adrenergic activity. The symptomatic effect of bromocriptine in Parkinson disease is attributed to its action at postsynaptic D_2 receptors in the striatum. Bromocriptine also inhibits the release of prolactin by a direct antagonist effect on the prolactin-secreting cells of the anterior pituitary. The prolactin-inhibiting effect of bromocriptine is the basis for its therapeutic effect in acromegaly and amenorrhea-galactorrhea.

Special Precautions

Bromocriptine may cause postural hypotension, particularly during the initiation of therapy. As such, its use in patients taking antihypertensive medication requires careful monitoring. This effect can be minimized by starting therapy with a bedtime dose before administering the drug.

There is no conclusive evidence that bromocriptine interacts with other ergot derivatives, but the combination of bromocriptine with other potential vasoconstrictors is not recommended.

Dosage

Parkinson's disease—Usual dosage range is from several milligrams to 40 mg daily. Object of initial dose is to establish tolerance. Intitial dose is 1.25 or 2.5 mg before bedtime, with food. Dose can subsequently be increased slowly by 1.25- or 2.5-mg increments in the total daily dose once weekly. *Hyperprolactinemia*—2.5 to 15 mg daily; *acromegaly*—20 to 60 mg.

IN BRIEF

Indications

Monotherapy in Parkinson's disease; adjunctive agent with other dopamine agonists, including levodopa; acromegaly; hyperprolactinemia

Adverse Effects

Nausea, constipation, orthostatic hypotension, postural hypotension leading to syncope, dyskinesias, confusion, agitation, hallucinations, drowsiness, light-headedness, nervousness, depression, anorexia, anxiety, mottling of skin, nasal congestion, nightmares, myoclonus

---

Rare: Signs of ergotism (tingling in the fingertips, digital vasospasm, Raynaud phenomenon, cold feet, muscle cramps in the legs and feet)

Pharmacokinetics and Pharmacodynamics

Elimination half-life: 2–8 h
Effect of food: adverse effects minimized or avoided by ingesting with food; absorption variable

Patient Information

Because bromocriptine is weaker than levodopa as a dopamine agonist, patients who do not respond to levodopa are not likely to benefit from bromocriptine. When bromocriptine is added to levodopa, the incidence of adverse effects may increase. Adverse effects may be reduced by temporarily decreasing the dosage of bromocriptine by 50% or more.

Availability

Tablets—2.5 mg
Capsules—5 mg

Carbidopa

(Lodosyn)

Carbidopa is a peripheral inhibitor of aromatic acid decarboxylase with its actions confined outside of the central nervous system. When given with levodopa, carbidopa prevents the peripheral decarboxylation and break-down of levodopa, enhancing its bioavailability and reducing nausea and other side effects that result from the stimulation by levodopa of periph-eral dopaminergic receptors. When taken alone, carbidopa has no overt pharmacodynamic actions. Carbidopa reduces by about 75% the amount of levodopa required to treat Parkinson's disease. It increases the plasma half-life of levodopa, increases plasma levodopa levels, and reduces the uri-nary excretion of levodopa and its metabolites. By blocking peripheral decarboxylase activity carbidopa prevents the effect of pyridoxine (vita-min B_6), which can inactivate levodopa by increasing the rate of the decar-boxylase enzyme. Thus, pyridoxine can be given to patients with Parkin-son's disease receiving levodopa when carbidopa is also taken.

Dosage

Whether given with pure levodopa or as a preparation that includes car-bidopa (*ie*, carbidopa-levodopa), dosage is determined by careful adjust-ment. Most patients respond to a 1:10 ratio of carbidopa-levodopa if the daily dose of carbidopa is 70 mg or more. The maximum daily dosage of carbidopa should not exceed 200 mg, but in practice, complete blockade of the peripheral decarboxylase enzyme may be achieved at lower doses. For a patient taking levodopa, carbidopa should be given as one 25-mg tablet three or four times daily, with levodopa. For patients experiencing nausea on regular or controlled-release carbidopa-levodopa preparations, carbidopa 25 mg may be given at the beginning of the day, simultaneously with the first dose of the carbidopa-levodopa preparation. Additional doses of half or one tablet may be given with subsequent doses of carbidopa-levodopa, as needed. The dosage of carbidopa may be adjusted by adding or omitting half or one tablet per day.

IN BRIEF

Indications

Levodopa-induced nausea and emesis

Adverse Effects

The only adverse reactions reported have occurred with concomitant levodopa or carbidopa-levodopa therapy. See adverse effects listed under levodopa.

Patient Information

Carbidopa does not decrease the central adverse effects of levodopa, such as hallucinations, off-fluctuations, and dyskinesias. In fact, by enabling more levodopa to reach the brain, carbidopa may enhance the potential of levodopa to induce these unwanted effects.

Availability

Tablets—25 mg

Clozapine
(*Clozaril*)

Clozapine is a tricyclic dibenzodiazepine derivative that has high potency in treating psychosis and yet has minimal central dopaminergic antagonism. Clozapine has a unique profile of receptor interactions, including D_4 receptor antagonism, serotonin receptor antagonism, α_2-receptor blockade, and partial M_1 cholinergic agonist activity. Clozapine appears to be more active at limbic dopamine receptors than at striatal dopamine receptors and, in contrast to conventional antipsychotics, does not induce parkinsonism or tardive dyskinesias. As such, clozapine has great potential in the treatment of psychosis and drug-induced hallucinations in patients with Parkinson's disease.

Clozapine is an effective antipsychotic agent for refractory schizophrenia. Clozapine also is indicated for the treatment of psychosis and hallucinations in Parkinson's disease. In the past, the development of hallucinations in Parkinson's disease patients taking levodopa or other agonists was treated only by reducing the dosage of the antiparkinsonian agents. Perhaps the greatest benefit conferred by clozapine is to allow Parkinson's disease patients with drug-induced hallucinations to continue taking their dopaminergic medication. There are several published reports of clozapine use in Parkinson's disease, consisting of open-label unblinded trials. Collectively, over 300 patients have been reported in this way, of whom over 80% had a successful result and were able to continue taking antiparkinsonian agents at the same or higher dose.

In reports of small numbers of patients, clozapine also has been reported to improve other movement disorders by a direct mechanism that is independent of the antipsychotic effect. These responses to clozapine include a reduction of parkinsonian tremor, improvement of levodopa-induced dyskinesias in Parkinson's disease, reduction of severe essential tremor, and improvement in dyskinesias and dystonia syndromes, including tardive dystonia [18]. Further trials are needed to establish the use of clozapine in these conditions.

The most frequent side effect in patients taking clozapine is dose-dependent sedation, which may remit with either continued therapy or dose reduction. The most serious potential adverse effect of clozapine is the induction of a severe idiosyncratic agranulocytosis, in as many as 1% of cases. Before intensive monitoring was instituted, this complication was related to at least 75 deaths in the United States. As a result, clozapine administration is now permitted only under the auspices of a unique surveillance arrangement, the Clozaril National Registry (1-800-448-5938). Patients must be assigned a registry number before they can take clozapine. Pharmacies are allowed to release only a 1 week supply at a time, and a weekly white blood cell count is required before the medication is renewed. The burden imposed on the patient and physician by the weekly monitoring requirement seems to be a necessary inconvenience. Since the monitoring system started, there has been no fatal case of clozapine-induced neutropenia in this country.

Special Precautions

Treatment with clozapine cannot be initiated in patients with white blood cell counts below 3500/mm^3.

Clozapine has anticholinergic activity and should be used with caution in patients with prostatism or narrow-angle glaucoma.

Clozapine may potentiate the effects of concurrently used anticholinergic agents.

Dosage

Begin with half or one tablet at night for 1 week, then slowly increase the dosage by half or one quarter tablet weekly. Daily doses of 25 to 100 mg have been shown to be sufficient to control severe hallucinations in Parkinson's disease.

IN BRIEF

Indications

Psychosis and hallucinations in Parkinson's disease

Contraindications

Myeloproliferative disorders, bone marrow suppressants, previous episode of neutropenia while taking clozapine

Adverse Effects

Dose-dependent sedation, dizziness, vertigo, headache, tremor, salivation, or dry mouth, visual disturbances, tachycardia, electrocardiographic changes, hypotension, syncope, constipation, nausea, severe idiosyncratic agranulocytosis

Pharmacokinetics and Pharmacodynamics

Peak action: 2.5 h
Plasma half-life: 8 h
Metabolism: almost entirely metabolized by liver

Patient Information

Parkinson's disease patients with hallucinations may be especially predisposed to the somnolence induced by clozapine. Orthostatic hypotension with or without syncope may occur at the start of clozapine therapy, especially with rapid dose escalation. Seizures have occurred in patients, apparently related to doses of clozapine exceeding 300 mg daily. The incidence of either acute dystonic reactions or the neuroleptic malignant syndrome is far lower than with conventional neuroleptics.

Availability

Tablets—25, 100 mg

Domperidone
(*Motilium*)

Domperidone is a peripheral dopamine antagonist structurally related to the butyrophenones. It has antiemetic and gastric prokinetic properties and is particularly useful in treating levodopa-induced nausea in Parkinson's disease. The mechanism of action is related to dopamine receptor blockade in the chemoreceptor trigger zone of the area postrema, outside the blood–brain barrier. Emesis induced by apomorphine, levodopa, and other drugs can be prevented by domperidone. There also may be a local antiemetic effect at the gastric mucosa. Because domperidone does not cross the blood–brain barrier, it has no central dopaminergic blocking effects and does not induce parkinsonism, tardive dyskinesias, or related complications.

Dosage

Usual dose is 1 to 2 tablets taken three or four times daily, 15 to 30 minutes before meals and before bedtime.

IN BRIEF

Indications

Levodopa-induced nausea in Parkinson's disease

Adverse Effects

Galactorrhea, gynecomastia, dry mouth, headaches, abdominal cramps; low incidence of side effects; <7%.

Pharmacokinetics and Pharmacodynamics

Peak action: IM—10–30 min; oral—30 min (taken on an empty stomach)
Plasma half-life: approximately 7 h

Availability

Tablets—10 mg

Levodopa
(Sinemet, Larodopa)

The introduction of levodopa replacement for Parkinson's disease followed pathologic and biochemical studies establishing that symptoms are due to selective loss of dopaminergic neurons in the substantia nigra. Levodopa therapy is the only treatment of a neurodegenerative disorder that provides a chemical precursor to replenish a deficient neurotransmitter. Although several dopamine agonists have been developed in the past three decades, none is more potent or effective than levodopa in treating Parkinson's disease. The synthetic pathway that produces dopamine begins with the amino acid tyrosine, which is converted to levodopa by the rate-limiting enzyme, tyrosine hydroxylase. Levodopa is decarboxylated to dopamine for release by presynaptic nerve terminals in the striatum. The synthetic output of this pathway cannot be increased by providing more substrate, tyrosine, because the rate of production is limited by tyrosine hydroxylase. Providing dopamine itself to a patient with Parkinson's disease also is ineffective because the neurotransmitter does not cross the blood–brain barrier to access the central nervous system. However, levodopa crosses the blood–brain barrier, and is converted to dopamine by brain dopa decarboxylase.

When levodopa is given orally, about 95% is decarboxylated in the gut, rendering the drug inactive for treating Parkinson's disease. To circumvent this problem, large doses of levodopa are required, or the drug must be given with a peripheral decarboxylase inhibitor. Several inhibitors are available, including carbidopa, which has been incorporated into the most widely used formulations of levodopa in North America, the levodopa-carbidopa combination.

Levodopa is the most potent agent for the symptomatic treatment of Parkinson's disease. It effectively reduces or abolishes all of the cardinal symptoms, particularly in mild or early cases. The response to levodopa is so predictable in most cases that clinicians view unequivocal benefit from this agent as diagnostic confirmation of Parkinson's disease. Idiopathic Parkinson's disease accounts for about 75% of all parkinsonism syndromes, and those who do not respond to even large doses of levodopa are generally considered to have atypical parkinsonism. Despite the efficacy of levodopa in Parkinson's disease, most clinicians do not use it as a first-line agent. It has never been established whether patients who receive levodopa replacement early in the course of Parkinson's disease have a different long-term result than those who postpone the use of levodopa. There is no consensus about the most appropriate time to initiate levodopa therapy in patients with mild to moderate parkinsonism. Postural instability, falling, festination, retropulsion, and gait-freezing are all indications for levodopa therapy, in efforts to prevent a serious fall. Moderately severe parkinsonism, corresponding to stage 3 of the Hoehn and Yahr scale or a decline in the capacity to carry out activities of daily living, are clear indications for levodopa treatment (Fig. 10-5).

Levodopa replacement may be associated with reversible adverse effects that may limit the therapy for Parkinson's disease. Among the commonest adverse effects of levodopa-carbidopa are gastrointestinal complaints. Nausea, anorexia, and vomiting are often reported, especially during the initiation of therapy. These problems are produced in large part by dopamine activation of the emesis center, the area postrema, lying outside of the blood–brain barrier. Peripheral decarboxylase inhibitors limit the peripheral formation of dopamine, a strategy that is highly effective in reducing nausea and emesis. These adverse effects also can be limited by having patients take levodopa-carbidopa with meals, increasing the dose gradually until tolerance develops, supplying additional carbidopa, using the controlled-release formulation of levodopa-carbidopa, or by adding the peripheral dopamine receptor antagonist, domperidone.

Central nervous system adverse effects are common in Parkinson's disease. Confusion, drowsiness, hypersomnolence, behavioral changes, vivid dreams, nightmares, or frank hallucinosis may follow levodopa treatment. The risk of these symptoms in some patients is often related to the dose of levodopa and to underlying dementia. These symptoms may be sufficiently disabling to warrant reduction in the dose of levodopa at the expense of worsening parkinsonism. Levodopa also can induce involuntary choreic movements, termed dyskinesias, in patients with parkinsonism. These movements are often mild but may increase in proportion to the dose of levodopa, necessitating reduction.

Dosage

Levodopa (Larodopa): Usual initial daily dosage is 500 to 1000 mg; dosage should not exceed 8000 mg daily. Levodopa is rarely prescribed alone because it is so likely to induce nausea and other side effects. The carbidopa-levodopa preparations are approximately four times more potent because of the peripheral decarboxylase inhibitor. A patient taking levodopa 1200 mg daily is receiving the equivalent dose of Sinemet 25/100 three times daily.

Carbidopa-levodopa preparations (Sinemet, Atamet): Combined tablets provide a carbidopa-to-levodopa ratio of 1:4 (Sinemet 25/100) and 1:10 (Sinemet 10/100 and 25/250). Patients should receive at least 70 to 100 mg daily of carbidopa. The usual starting dose for symptomatic therapy is about 300 mg of the levodopa component. Hence, typical starting regimen is carbidopa-levodopa (Sinemet) 25/100 three times daily.

Long-acting controlled-release preparations of carbidopa-levodopa (Sinemet CR 25/100 and Sinemet CR 50/200): Provide a sustained-release matrix allowing delivery of carbidopa and levodopa for 4 to 6 hours. Controlled-release preparations have a slower onset of effect, less bioavailability, and longer duration of effect than regular carbidopa-levodopa preparations. The peak concentration of levodopa occurs 2 hours after ingestion of the controlled-release preparation, as opposed to 30 minutes or less for regular carbidopa-levodopa.

Hoehn and Yahr rating scale for Parkinson's Disease	
Stage 1	Mild, unilateral Parkinson's disease
Stage 2	Bilateral symptoms, without balance impairment
Stage 3	Postural instability, but physically independent
Stage 4	Severely disabled but still able to walk or stand assisted
Stage 5	Wheelchair-bound or bedridden unless aided

FIGURE 10-5 Hoehn and Yahr rating scale for Parkinson's disease. (*From* Hoehn and colleague (19); with permission.)

IN BRIEF

Indications
Symptomatic treatment of Parkinson's disease

Adverse Effects
Nausea, anorexia, vomiting, confusion, drowsiness, hypersomnolence, behavioral changes, vivid dreams, nightmares, frank hallucinosis, postural hypotension, cardiac arrhythmias

Pharmacokinetics and Pharmacodynamics
Peak action: 30–90 min; peak brain levels reached 1 h later

Patient Information
Gastrointestinal adverse effects can be limited by having patients take levodopa and carbidopa with meals, increasing the dose gradually until tolerance develops, supplying additional carbidopa, using the controlled-release formulation of levodopa and carbidopa, or by adding the peripheral dopamine receptor antagonist domperidone. Postural hypotension can be helped by increasing fluid and salt intake, the use of antigravity stockings, and the administration of fludrocortisone or midodrine.

Availability
Levodopa: Tablets—100, 250, 500 mg
Carbidopa-levodopa preparations: Tablets—25 mg carbidopa/100 mg levodopa, 10 mg carbidopa/100 mg levodopa
Controlled-release preparations: Tablets—CR 25/100, CR 50/200

Pergolide
(Permax)

Pergolide mesylate is a synthetic ergot derivative that acts as a potent dopamine agonist at D_2 receptors and a weak agonist at D_1 receptors. In Parkinson's disease, pergolide is believed to exert a therapeutic effect by directly stimulating postsynaptic dopaminergic receptors in the striatum. Its dopamine agonist potency exceeds by about tenfold that of bromocriptine on a milligram per milligram basis.

Special Precautions

Pergolide may cause hypotension in susceptible patients and should be administered with appropriate caution. Concurrent use of antihypertensive medication may exacerbate this effect. As such, it is best to warn patients about this possibility, begin treatment with a small dose, and increase the dosage slowly over several weeks.

Hypotension leading to syncope has occurred in patients, usually at the initiation of therapy. Gradual dosage adjustment usually leads to resolution of this problem.

Pergolide should be given with caution to patients with cardiac disease. In a study comparing pergolide and placebo, patients taking pergolide were found to experience a significantly higher incidence of atrial arrhythmias.

The abrupt discontinuation of pergolide may trigger hallucinosis and confusion with an acute exacerbation of parkinsonism. Discontinuation of the drug should be done gradually, even if the patient is to remain on levodopa.

Dosage

Initiate pergolide treatment with a single daily dose of 0.05 mg for the first several days, gradually increasing thereafter by 0.1 to 0.15 mg every third day for the next 2 weeks. If tolerated, pergolide can be increased in 0.25 mg increments every third day to the optimal dosage, as determined by symptom relief and presence of adverse effects. Safety of dosages more than 5 mg/d has not been evaluated.

IN BRIEF

Indications

Symptomatic therapy for Parkinson's disease, as adjunct to levodopa treatment or monotherapy

Adverse Effects

Central nervous system symptoms, including dyskinesias, somnolence, and hallucinations; nausea; constipation; diarrhea; dyspepsia; hypotension; rhinitis

Pharmacokinetics and Pharmacodynamics

Onset of action: 15–30 min
Peak action: 1–2 h

Patient Information

Some adverse effects of pergolide, such as dyskinesias and hallucinations, occurred in people who were taking levodopa and other dopamine agonists, agents that also may cause these side effects. These adverse effects can be reduced by decreasing the dose of pergolide, levodopa, or other concurrent medication.

Availability

Tablets—0.05, 0.25, 1 mg

Selegiline
(Deprenyl, Eldepryl)

Selegiline is a synthetic, selective, irreversible inhibitor of monoamine oxidase type B, a catalytic enzyme for dopamine. The agent is an antioxidant, and its use in Parkinson's disease is aimed at slowing the progression of the condition. The cause of Parkinson's disease has not been discovered, although oxidation injury to nigral neurons may contribute. The rationale for the use of selegiline is that reduction of oxidation injury may retard the loss of substantia nigra neurons. In 400 patients receiving selegiline 10 mg/d in a large, multicenter, randomized, placebo-controlled trial, the need for instituting levodopa replacement therapy was delayed by about 9 months (Fig. 10-6) [20]. Selegiline may delay the need for symptomatic treatment of Parkinson's disease, but it also appears to have its own mild symptomatic effect on the disease. The actual effect of selegiline in Parkinson's disease may be the sum of several processes, including both symptomatic and neuroprotective mechanisms.

Special Precautions

In doses exceeding 10 mg daily, the selectivity of selegiline for the monoamine oxidase type B enzyme declines, and the agent may inhibit both monoamine oxidase types A and B. As such, selegiline may present the same possible adverse effect profile as the monoamine oxidase type A drugs, which include hypotension and other symptoms of catecholamine deficiency.

In theory, selegiline in high dose can precipitate a state of excessive catecholamine function, the so-called hypertensive crisis, if it is taken with tyramine-containing substances, such as red wine and aged cheese. Similarly, the combination of high-dose selegiline and serotonin reuptake inhibitors commonly prescribed for depression may precipitate a serotonin syndrome.

Dosage

Usual dosage is one tablet twice daily, taken at breakfast and lunch time. Taking selegiline in the late afternoon or evening is thought to render more likely the adverse effect of insomnia. Doses higher than 10 mg daily should not be used.

IN BRIEF

Indications
First-line drug in mild Parkinson's disease to delay the introduction of levodopa, weak symptomatic agent in combination with levodopa-carbidopa

Adverse Effects
Exacerbation of levodopa-induced adverse effects, such as dyskinesias; neurobehavioral disturbances, such as nightmares, insomnia, confusion, and hallucinations

Availability
Tablets—5 mg

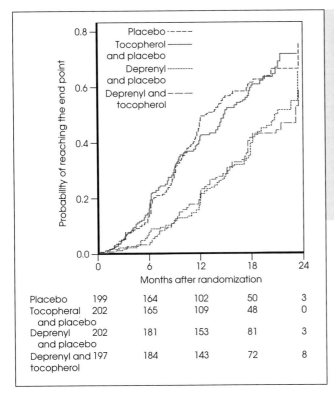

Placebo	199	164	102	50	3
Tocopheral and placebo	202	165	109	48	0
Deprenyl and placebo	202	181	153	81	3
Deprenyl and tocopherol	197	184	143	72	8

FIGURE 10-6 Kaplan-Meier curves depicting the probability of reaching the endpoint at which levodopa therapy is required in patients with early Parkinson's disease. The number of patients in each group is listed below the graph. During the study period, patients taking deprenyl were less likely to require levodopa therapy. Tocopherol, or vitamin E, had no effect on Parkinson's disease. (*From the Parkinson's Study Group (20); with permission.*)

Baclofen
(Lioresal)

Baclofen is a direct agonist of the $GABA_B$ type receptors located throughout the central nervous system, with a high concentration in the superficial layers of the spinal cord. The drug is a muscle relaxant used primarily in the treatment of spasticity and is discussed more fully elsewhere. It also has a weak nociceptive effect, making it a potentially useful medication in pain syndromes and in conditions characterized by painful cramping. Baclofen is also a first-line drug in the treatment of many movement disorders, particularly dystonia.

Dosage

Dystonia: Dosages of 40 to 80 mg daily represent the average range, but resistant or severe cases may require dosages of 120 or 150 mg daily, or more.

IN BRIEF

Indications
Dystonia; spasticity of spinal origin

Adverse Effects
Most common: Dose-dependent nausea and drowsiness

Availability
Tablets—10, 20 mg

Botulinum toxin A
(Occulinum)

Botulinum toxin injections provide a unique therapeutic modality in patients with focal movement disorders, notably focal dystonia and hemifacial spasm [21]. The toxin is produced by the anaerobic bacterium *Clostridium botulinum* and is responsible for botulism. Seven immunologically distinct serotypes are distinguished, A to G. Botulinum toxin serotypes A, B, and F have therapeutic usefulness, but only botulinum toxin A is presently available. Botulinum toxin exerts a paralytic action at the neuromuscular junction by inhibiting the release of acetylcholine from the presynaptic nerve terminal. Following an intramuscular injection of botulinum toxin, the muscle becomes denervated, developing weakness and atrophy. At the microscopic level, the process of denervation begins within hours of the injection, but the clinical effect usually develops between 2 and 10 days afterward. The degree and duration of effect of botulinum toxin depend on the severity of the movement disorder and the quantity of toxin injected, assuming optimal injection technique. Most patients receiving botulinum toxin derive clinical benefit for an average of 3 months.

Dosage

Botulinum toxin injections for dystonia should be performed only by physicians who are familiar with dystonia, other movement disorders, and the anatomy of the region being injected, and who have basic electromyogram (EMG) skills. Botulinum toxin is injected into muscles through a hollow needle or electrode (Fig. 10-7). Although the target muscles can be identified easily in injections for blepharospasm or most cases of torticollis, EMG recording helps to identify the muscles involved in complex dystonic movements. Cervical dystonia may involve combinations of different movements, or there may be a tremor. Under these circumstances, EMG is used for precise localization by means of a hollow-tipped needle electrode through which the toxin can be injected. Injections of the vocal cords in spasmodic dysphonia also should be performed using EMG guidance.

IN BRIEF

Indications

Blepharospasm, spasmodic dysphonia, oromandibular dystonia, cervical dystonia, focal dystonia of the limbs, facial tics, hemifacial spasm

Adverse Effects

Excessive muscle weakness at the injection site, resulting in ptosis, watery eyes, or dry eyes as complications of blepharospasm treatment; neck weakness and dysphagia as complications of torticollis treatment; hypophonia as a complication of vocal cord treatment; excessive hand weakness as a complication of focal hand dystonia treatment; pain and tenderness at the injection site; transient flu-like illness characterized by myalgia and malaise.

Patient Information

A small percentage of patients exposed to repeated injections of botulinum toxin may develop resistance to the beneficial effect, with no muscle weakness, atrophy, or improvement following an injection. In some of these people, serum antibodies to botulinum toxin can be detected using a mouse lethality assay. The incidence of this complication of therapy, estimated at 10%, can be reduced by limiting the dose or frequency of injection, although no clear guidelines are completely effective.

Availability

Freeze-dried concentrate reconstituted in saline. Vials—100 units of toxin, as determined using a mouse lethality assay (LD_{50}); concentration of 2.5, 5, or 10 units/0.1 mL

Movement Disorder	Muscle	Average Starting Dose	Usual Dose Range (U)
Blepharospasm	Orbicularis oculi	20	15–100
Hemificial spasm	Orbicularis oculi	12.5	10–25
	Facial muscles	2.5	1.25–5
Blinking tics	Orbicularis oculi	12.5	12.5–25
Oromandibular dystonia	Masseter	25	10–75
	Temporalis	20	5–50
	Medial pterygoid	20	5–40
	Lateral pterygoid	20	5–40
Meige syndrome—craniofacial dystonia	Zygomaticus	5	2.5–7.5
	Risorius	5	2.5–10
Spasmodic dysphonia	Thyroarytenoid	1.8	12.5–5
Torticollis	Sternocleidomastoid	25	12.5–50
	Trapezius	80	25–200
	Levator scapula	50	10–80
	Splenius	50	20–100
	Scalene muscles	20	10–60
Limb dystonia*	Hand (intrinsic hand muscles)	7.5	2.5–12.5
	Arm	30	5–45
	Foot (intrinsic foot muscles)	60	35–85
	Leg	85	45–125
Trunk	–	85	50–120

* Botulinum toxin doses listed for limb and trunk dystonia represent the combined total units for each body part, not individual muscles. Botulinum toxin A doses for facial and neck muscles and vocal cords derived from the botulinum toxin computerized database at the Center for Movement Disorders, Columbia–Presbyterian Medical Center. Doses for limb muscles provided by Dr. Seth Pullman, Clinical Motor Physiology Laboratory, Columbia Medical Center.

FIGURE 10-7

Dosage recommendations for botulinum toxin A intramuscular injections used in the treatment of movement disorders.

Clonidine
(Catapres)

Clonidine is a centrally acting α-adrenergic receptor agonist with complex actions at presynaptic and postsynaptic receptor sites. In the peripheral nervous system, clonidine decreases adrenergic transmission by activating presynaptic α_2 receptors. Clonidine, initially employed as a nasal decongestant, is primarily used as an antihypertensive agent. Clonidine is effective in the treatment for tic disorders.

Special Precautions

The sudden discontinuation of clonidine may precipitate a rebound adrenergic discharge, resulting in a hypertensive crisis.

Dosage

Dosage range for Tourette syndrome is identical to that for hypertension, 0.2 to 0.8 mg daily, in two or more divided doses.

IN BRIEF

Indications
Tic disorders

Adverse Effects
Dry mouth, drowsiness, dizziness, nausea, indigestion, impotence, vivid dreams or nightmares, insomnia, restlessness, anxiety, depression

Availability
Tablets—0.1, 0.2, 0.3 mg

Penicillamine
(Cuprimine)

Penicillamine is 3-mercapto-D-valine, a chelating agent effective for the removal of excess copper in Wilson's disease. Two molecules of penicillamine can bind 1 atom of copper, and 1 g of penicillamine can theoretically chelate 200 mg of copper. The copper mobilized by penicillamine is excreted by the kidneys. Treatment of Wilson's disease can be divided into initial and maintenance phases. The initial phase is directed at reducing the body copper excess to a subtoxic level, which usually requires 4 to 6 months of treatment. Improvement in neurologic symptoms often does not begin until 6 months after the copper is reduced and may continue for several years. Maintenance therapy follows the initial decoppering phase and is directed at preventing the recurrence of copper toxicity. Treatment is mandatory for the rest of the patient's life.

Special Precautions

The potential for a serious renal or hematologic complication at any time requires careful surveillance. During the first 6 months of penicillamine therapy, it is recommended to obtain a urinalysis and complete blood count every 2 weeks. After the first 6 months of therapy, routine screening tests can be performed every month or less frequently.

In pregnancy, penicillamine therapy should be continued to protect the mother from a relapse of Wilson's disease.

Dosage

To permit maximum absorption, the medication should be taken on an empty stomach, at least 1 hour before meals or 2 hours after meals. The initial dose is 250 mg daily, gradually increasing over 2 weeks to 1000 mg daily, usually given in 2 or 4 divided doses. Initially, this dose of penicillamine induces an abundant cupriuresis, but this effect gradually tapers as the excess body copper accumulation is gradually depleted. The maintenance dose of penicillamine is usually the same as the initial dose. Penicillamine is administered with pyridoxine 20 mg daily to prevent the vitamin B_6 deficiency that the chelating agent may induce.

IN BRIEF

Indications

Symptomatic Wilson's disease, prevention of neurologic and hepatic symptoms in patients with asymptomatic Wilson's disease

Adverse Effects

Short-term: Hypersensitivity in the form of a fulminant febrile reaction, exacerbation of Wilson's disease symptoms

Long-term: Fever, skin rashes, lymphadenopathy, gastrointestinal symptoms, decreased taste sensation; leukopenia, thrombocytopenia, proteinuria, hematuria, systemic lupus erythematosus, polyarthritis, optic neuritis, Goodpasture syndrome, myasthenic syndrome sometimes progressing to myasthenia gravis

Prolonged Use

The efficacy of chelation therapy is determined by measurement of a 24-h copper excretion. In the first week of penicillamine therapy, a dose resulting in a 24-h excretion rate of 2 mg of copper should be continued for at least 3 mo. Gradually the 24-h urine copper declines to <500 µg, and in the maintenance phase, <150 µg/24 h. The most useful test in assessing efficacy of treatment after the initial phase is the serum free copper determination, which in adequately treated patients is <10 µg/dL. Adherence to a strict low-copper diet in Wilson's disease is not mandatory, but avoidance of certain high copper-containing foods, such as liver and shellfish, is advised.

Patient Information

Drug fever, usually in the second or third week following initiation of therapy, may necessitate a reduction in the penicillamine dose or temporary cessation of treatment. Pretreatment with corticosteroids may be helpful in reducing this complication.

Availability

Capsules—125, 250 mg

Reserpine

Reserpine is one member of a class of medications known as rauwolfia alkaloids, derived from plant extracts, which have been used for centuries. Reserpine is a catecholamine depletor that interferes with the intracellular stores of central nervous system catecholamines, including dopamine. The pharmacologic effect may be irreversible because reaccumulation of catecholamine requires the formation of new synaptic storage vesicles. Historically the most common indications for reserpine have been treatment of hypertension and psychosis. The availability of better tolerated antihypertensives and antipsychotics has greatly reduced use of reserpine, and the drug is becoming difficult to obtain. In the treatment of movement disorders, however, reserpine has a unique and potent ability to suppress various hyperkinetic movement disorders, such as tics, chorea, dyskinesias, and tardive dystonia.

Special Precautions

Reserpine has been linked epidemiologically to risk of breast carcinoma.

The drug is difficult to titrate because of a long duration of action.

There is a lag time between a dose change and clinical effect, making difficult a precise interpretation of the drug effect.

Reserpine is often combined with other antihypertensive agents, such as hydrochlorothiazide. Combination forms have limited usefulness in the treatment of movement disorders because they needlessly reduce the blood pressure.

Dosage

Starting dose should be half or one tablet at bedtime for a week, with gradual increases in the dose each week subsequently. Careful monitoring for hypotension, depression, and sedation should be done as long as the patient takes the medication. The usual range for hypertension is 0.1 to 1 mg daily, but in severe movement disorders, daily doses as high as 3 to 8 mg have been employed safely and with good effect.

IN BRIEF

Indications
Tics, chorea, dyskinesias, tardive dystonia

Contraindications
Depression, hypotension

Adverse Effects
Somnolence, hypotension, vivid dreams, insomnia, depression, parkinsonism

Availability
Tablets—0.25 mg

Pramipexole
(Mirapex)

Pramipexole is the first of a new generation of non-ergot dopamine agonists for use in treating Parkinson's disease, released in the United States in July 1997. Other new compounds in this family include ropinerole and cabergoline. Pramipexole is a D_2 agonist that has additional agonist activity at D_3 receptor sites, located in the ventral striatum (nucleus accumbens) and olfactory tubercle [22]. The relevance of D_3 receptor binding in Parkinson's disease is unknown, but because the drug is not an ergot derivative, it is hoped that the incidence of side effects will be less than that associated with the earlier dopamine agonists bromocriptine and pergolide. The efficacy of pramipexole is similar to that of bromocriptine and pergolide when given in optimal and equivalent dosage. On a milligram basis, the dopamine agonist potency is approximately that of pergolide.

There is little clinical experience to date with pramipexole, outside of clinical trials. Trials of pramipexole as monotherapy in early Parkinson's disease showed symptomatic relief as compared to placebo. In advanced Parkinson's disease, when pramipexole was added to levodopa, pramipexole was associated with improvements in motor function, decreased disability, and reduction in wearing-off fluctuations [23]. Pramipexole also enabled a decrease in the daily levodopa requirement [23].

Special Precautions

Pramipexole is secreted 90% unchanged in the urine. As such, patients with renal disease require lower doses of pramipexole. Pramipexole may potentiate the dopaminergic adverse effects of levodopa and other dopamine agonists when used concurrently.

Dosage

Like all dopamine agonists, pramipexole should be started at a subtherapeutic dose and be gradually titrated upwards over several weeks to full effectiveness. The titration schedule must be modified if adverse effects develop. The starting dose is 0.125 mg three times a day, gradually increasing by increments of 50% to 100% each week over 4 to 8 weeks, reaching a maximum daily dose of 4 to 6 mg, in three divided doses. The dosage is reduced in the presence of renal disease, as indicated in the package insert. In clinical trials, daily doses of 1.5 to 4.5 mg were well-tolerated by patients, even when given with as much as 800 mg levodopa daily.

IN BRIEF

Indications

Symptomatic therapy as a single agent in early idiopathic Parkinson's disease, or in conjunction with levodopa in more advanced Parkinson's disease

Adverse Effects

The commonest adverse effects of pramipexole when given as a single agent in early Parkinson's disease in clinical trials were excessive drowsiness, nausea, dizziness, hallucinations, constipation, and hypotension. When given with levodopa to patients with more advanced Parkinson's disease, pramipexole was associated with dyskinesias and hallucinations.

Pharmacokinetics and Pharmacodynamics

Peak action: 2 h
Half-life: 8 h

Availability

Tablets—0.125, 0.25, 1.0, 1.5 mg

Olanzapine

(*Zyprexa*)

Olanzapine is an antipsychotic agent of the thiobenzodiazepine class. Pharmacologically, olanzapine is an antagonist at several brain receptors, including serotonin 5HT, dopamine (D_1 to D_4), muscarinic, histaminic, and α-1 adrenergic. Like clozapine, olanzapine is an atypical neuroleptic with a low incidence of extrapyramidal adverse effects, including drug-induced parkinsonism. As such, it is a useful agent for the treatment of psychosis and hallucinosis in patients with Parkinson's disease. Unlike clozapine, olanzapine is not associated with drug-induced neutropenia, and therefore does not require weekly white blood cell count monitoring. Its convenience of use relative to clozapine makes olanzapine a potentially valuable agent in Parkinson patients with psychosis.

In an open-label trial involving 15 non-demented patients with Parkinson's disease and drug-induced psychosis, treatment with olanzapine reduced psychosis and did not cause an increase in parkinsonism, according to rating scales [24]. The mean daily dose of olanzapine was 6.5 mg, ranging between 2 to 15 mg. Olanzapine also induced a significant increase in total sleep time, suggesting a potential use as an hypnotic agent in Parkinson's disease. The effect of long-term olanzapine treatment in patients with Parkinson's disease is not known, and will require longer clinical experience.

Special Precautions

The most serious potential adverse effects of olanzapine are neuroleptic malignant syndrome and tardive dyskinesia. Neither has been described with olanzapine, but clinical experience is still too limited to know the incidence of these rare complications. In pre-clinical trials involving a total of 2500 patients with schizophrenia, there was a higher incidence of restlessness, or akathisia, in patients taking olanzapine, as compared to placebo, especially at daily doses exceeding 5 mg. The incidence of drug-induced parkinsonism or dyskinesias did not differ between olanzapine and placebo. However, in clinical practice at the Center for Parkinson's Disease, Columbia-Presbyterian Medical Center, several patients who were switched from clozapine to olanzapine reported an unacceptable increase in parkinsonism. This suggests the dopamine antagonist activity of olanzapine exceeds that of clozapine and can be clinically significant.

Dosage

The recommended starting dose in Parkinson's disease is 5 mg at bedtime. The dose can be increased by 5 mg each week to a target dose of 10 mg or 15 mg, if needed. The safety of daily doses exceeding 20 mg has not been evaluated.

IN BRIEF

Indications

Psychosis and hallucinosis in Parkinson's disease

Adverse Effects

Like clozapine, olanzapine may induce orthostatic hypotension and excessive somnolence. In pre-clinical trials, the most commonly noted adverse effects included constipation, dry mouth, cognitive impairment, weight gain, hyper-prolactinemia, peripheral edema, and an elevation in liver transaminases.

Pharmacokinetics and Pharmacodynamics

Peak Effect 6 h after oral dose
Half-life: 30 h

Availability

Tablets—5, 7.5, 10 mg

Ropinerole

(Requip)

Ropinerole is the second of a new generation of non-ergoline dopamine agonists that binds to the post synaptic D_2 family of receptors, comprising D_2, D_3, and D_4 receptors. In this respect, it would appear to share a similar binding profile as pramipexole, the other non-ergoline dopamine agonist. Ropinerole has little activity at D_1 receptors, unlike pergolide or bromocriptine. Its symptomatic effect in Parkinson's disease (PD) is attributed to D_2 agonist effects at the receptors in the caudate and putamen.

Ropinerole is effective as monotherapy in early PD, or as an adjuvant agent in patients with advanced PD taking levodopa. In a multicenter, randomized placebo-controlled clinical trial, ropinerole monotherapy for patients with mild PD improved Unified Parkinson's Disease Rating Scale (UPDRS) motor scores and was well-tolerated [25]. The mean daily ropinerole dose in this study was approximately 15 mg. In an unpublished comparison of ropinerole (mean daily dose 12 mg) to bromocriptine (mean daily dose 24 mg) in the treatment of early PD, ropinerole was more effective in reducing parkinsonian motor scores on the UPDRS. When added to levodopa in patients with advanced PD complicated by wearing-off fluctuations, ropinerole was associated with a mean reduction in "off" time of 1 hour daily, and a reduction in levodopa daily dose requirement by about 20% [26].

Dosing

The recommended starting dose is 0.25 mg three times a day, with upward titration in weekly 0.25 mg dose increments to 1 mg three times a day within 4 weeks, as required. After the 4th week, the dose may be increased by a daily dose of 1.5 mg each week to 9 mg daily, and then by 3 mg per day weekly to a total dose of 24 mg daily.

IN BRIEF

Indications

Monotherapy in early Parkinson's disease, or as an adjuvant agent in patients with advanced PD taking levodopa

Pharmacokinetics

Ropinerole reaches peak serum concentration 1 to 2 hours after an oral dose. Ropinerole is extensively metabolized by the liver to inactive metabolites. Its elimination half-life is 6 hours.

Adverse Effects

The most common side effect is nausea, occurring in as many as half the patients who received ropinerole in one study, but it was rarely severe enough to warrant discontinuation. This adverse effect can be reduced by taking the medication with food. Dizziness and somnolence are also frequent. Other less common side effects include headache, syncope, edema, fatigue, hallucinations, and confusion. When taken in tandem with levodopa, drug-induced dyskinesias are common, but can also occur with ropinerole as monotherapy.

Availability

Tablets 0.25, 0.5, 1.0, 2.0, 5.0 mg

Tolcapone

(Tasmar)

Tolcapone is an inhibitor of cathechol-O-methyl transferase (COMT), an enzyme that catalyzes the methylation of levodopa to its metabolite 3-O-methyldopa (3-OMD). This metabolic reaction diverts a portion of the levodopa supply from conversion to dopamine. A COMT inhibitor prevents or limits this "metabolic loss" of levodopa to 3-OMD, increasing its availability for dopamine production. COMT also metabolizes dopamine to 3-methoxytyramine (3-MT) and the dopamine metabolite dihydroxphenylacetic acid (DOPAC) to homovanillic acid (HVA) (Fig. 10-8).

Tolcapone is a selective, reversible, peripherally and centrally active COMT inhibitor. Thirty minutes after oral administration, tolcapone suppresses liver and brain COMT activity by about 70% [27]. Full recovery of COMT activity is attained 16 hours after a single oral dose. When taken in combination with levodopa and a peripheral dopa decarboxylase inhibitor, such as carbidopa or benserazide, tolcapone prevents the breakdown of levodopa to 3-OMD in the gut, enabling more levodopa to enter the bloodstream and eventually cross the blood-brain barrier (Fig. 10-8). As such, tolcapone increases the bioavailability and plasma levels of levodopa and prolongs its half-life. Tolcapone also enters the brain directly, where it increases whole brain concentrations of levodopa and dopamine, and reduces the levels of metabolites 3-OMD, 3-MT, and HVA.

The primary role for tolcapone in Parkinson's disease is an adjunct agent for use with levodopa, levodopa/carbidopa, or levodopa/benserazide. In clinical trials to date, tolcapone prolonged the antiparkinsonian effect of levodopa when taken with a peripheral decarboxylase inhibitor [28]. In patients with end-of-levodopa-dose wearing-off effects, tolcapone

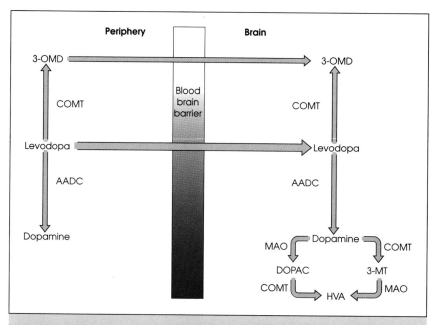

FIGURE 10-8 Metabolism of levodopa. AADC—Aromatic amino acid decarboxylase; COMT—catechol-O-methyl transferase; DOPAC—dihydroxyphenylacetic acid; HVA—homovanillic acid; MAO—monoamine oxidase; 3-MT—3-methoxytyramine; 3-OMD—3-O-methyldopa. (*Adapted from* Mannisto (30); with permission.)

improved motor function and reduced off fluctuations [29]. Tolcapone accentuated levodopa-induced dyskinesias in the clinical trials, necessitating a reduction in the daily levodopa dosage.

Because tolcapone can potentiate the therapeutic effects of levodopa, it may be especially useful for the patient taking levodopa who experiences wearing-off fluctuations. Alternative treatments for this problem include shortening the levodopa dosing interval, using a controlled release levodopa preparation, or adding a dopamine agonist. Tolcapone can also increase the adverse effects of levodopa, such as levodopa-induced dyskinesias. Because it is a new drug, more clinical experience is needed to know how tolcapone, and the concept of COMT inhibition will fit into the therapeutic repertoire for Parkinson's disease.

Dosage

Starting dose is 50 mg three times a day, taken with levodopa/carbidopa or levodopa/benserazide, increasing if needed to a maximum dose of 400 mg three times a day.

IN BRIEF

Indications
Adjunct agent for use with levodopa in the symptomatic treatment of Parkinson's disease

Adverse Effects
Diarrhea, nausea, postural hypotension, dizziness, urine discoloration, and prolongation and increase of levodopa-induced adverse effects, including dyskinesias

Pharmacokinetics and Pharamacodynamics
Onset of effect is 30 min after oral administration, causing COMT suppression by about 70%. Full recovery of COMT activity occurs 16 h after a single oral dose.

Availability
Tablets—50, 200, 400 mg

References

1. Lang AE, Weiner W: *Movement Disorders: A Comprehensive Survey.* Mount Kisco, NY: Futura; 1989.
2. Albin R, Young AB, Penney JB: The functional anatomy of basal ganglia disorders. *Trends Neurosci* 1989, 12:366–375.
3. Cooper JR, Bloom FE, Roth RH: *The Biochemical Basis of Neuropharmacology*, edn 5. New York: Oxford University Press; 1986.
4. Koller WC, Silver DE, Lieberman A: An algorithm for the management of Parkinson's disease. *Neurology* 1994, 44(suppl 10):5–52.
5. Burke RE, Fahn S, Marsden CD: Torsion dystonia: a double blind, prospective trial of high dose trihexyphenidyl. *Neurology* 1986, 36:160–164.
6. Cedarbaum JM, Schleifer LS: Drugs for Parkinson's disease, spasticity and acute muscle spasm. In *The Pharmacological Basis of Therapeutics*, edn 8. Edited by Goodman AG, Rall TW, Nies AW, Taylor P. New York: Pergamon; 1990:477.
7. Golbe LI, Sage JI: Medical treatment of Parkinson's disease. In *Treatment of Movement Disorders*. Edited by Kurlan R. Philadelphia: JB Lippincott; 1995:1–56.
8. Jankovic J, Mardsen CD: Therapeutic strategies in Parkinson's disease. In *Parkinson's Disease and Movement Disorders*, edn 2. Edited by Jankovic J, Tolosa E. Baltimore: Williams & Wilkins; 1993:116.
9. Kurth MC, Tetrud JW, Irwin I, *et al.*: Oral levodopa/carbidopa solution versus tablets in Parkinson's disease with severe fluctuations: a pilot study. *Neurology* 1993, 43:1036–1039.

10. Kurth MC, Tetrud JW, Tanner CM, *et al.*: Double-blind, placebo-controlled, crossover study of duodenal infusion of levodopa/carbidopa in Parkinson's disease patients with 'on-off' fluctuations. *Neurology* 1993, 43:1698–1703.

11. Roberts JW, Cora-Locateli G, Bravi D, *et al.*: Catechol-O-methyltransferase inhibitor tolcapone prolongs levodopa/carbidopa action in parkinsonian patients. *Neurology* 1994, 44:2685–2688.

12. Bennett JP Jr, Landow ER, Schuh LA: Suppression of dyskinesis in advanced Parkinson's disease: increasing daily clozapine doses supress dyskinesia and improve parkinsonism symptoms. *Neurology* 1993, 42:1551–1555.

13. Schuh LA, Bennett JP Jr: Suppression of dyskinesias in advanced Parkinson's disease: continuous intravenous levodopa shifts dose response for production of dyskinesias but not for relief of parkinsonism in patients with advanced Parkinson's disease. *Neurology* 1993, 43:1545–1550.

14. Greene P, Shale H, Fahn S: Analysis of open-label trials in torsion dystonia using high dosages of anticholingerics and other drugs. *Movement Disorders* 1998, 13:402.

15. Kang U, Burke RE, Fahn S: Natural history and treatment of tardive dystonia. *Movement Disorders* 1986, 1:193–208.

16. Brewer GJ, Yuzbasiyan-Gurkan V: Wilson disease. *Medicine* 1992, 71:139–164.

17. Frankel JP, Lees AJ, Kempster PA, *et al.*: Subcutaneous apomorphine in the treatment of Parkinson's disease. *J Neurol Neurosurg Psychiatr* 1990, 53:96.

18. Lieberman JA, Saltz BL, Johns CA, *et al.*: Effects of clozapine on tardive dyskinesia. *Br J Psychiatr* 1991, 158:503–510.

19. Hoehn MM, Yahr MD: Parkinsonism: onset, progression and mortality. *Neurology* 1967, 17:427–442.

20. The Parkinson's Study Group: Effects of tocopherol and deprenyl on the progression of disability in early Parkinson's disease. *N Engl J Med* 1993, 328:176.

21. Jankovic J, Hallet M: *Botulinum Toxin Treatment.* New York: Marcel Dekker, 1994.

22. Piercey MF, Walker EL, Feldpaush DL, Camacho-Ochoa M: High affinity binding for pramipexole, a dopamine D3 receptor ligand, in rat striatum. *Neurosci Lett* 1996, 219:138–140.

23. Lieberman A, Ranhosky A, Korts D: Clinical evaluation of pramipexole in advanced Parkinson's disease. *Neurology* 1997, 49:162-168.

24. Wolters EC, Jansen ENH, Tuynman-Qua HG, Bergmans PLM: Olanzapine in the treatment of dopaminomimetic psychosis in patients with Parkinson's disease. *Neurology* 1996, 46:1085–1087.

25. Adler CH, Sethi KD, Davis TL, Hammerstad JP, *et al.*: Ropinerole for the treatment of early Parkinson's disease. *Neurology* 1997, 49:393–399.

26. Kreider MS, Knox S, Gardiner D, *et al.*: A multicenter double blind study of ropinerole as an adjunct to L-dopa in Parkinson's disease. *Neurology* 1996, 46:A475 [abstract].

27. Kaakkola S, Gordin A, Mannisto PT: General properties and clinical possibilities of new selective inhibitors of catechol-O-methyltransferase. *Gen Pharmacol* 1994, 25:813–824.

28. Roberts JW, Cora-Locatelli G, Bravi D, *et al.*: Catechol-O-methyltransferase inhibitor tolcapone prolongs levodopa/carbidopa action in parkinsonian patients. *Neurology* 1994, 44:2685–2688.

29. Kurth MC, Adler CH, St. Hilaire M, Singer C, *et al.*: Tolcapone improves motor function and reduces levodopa requirement in patients with Parkinson's disease experiencing motor fluctuations. *Neurology* 1997, 48:81–87.

30. Mannisto PT: Clinical potential of catechol-O-methyltransferase inhibitors as adjuvants in Parkinson's disease. *CNS Drugs* 1994, 1:172–179.

Index

Color Plates

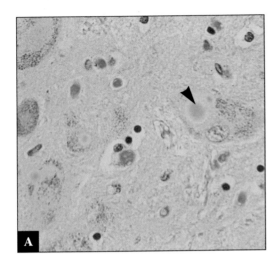

Chapter 2, Figure 2-7A, p. 21

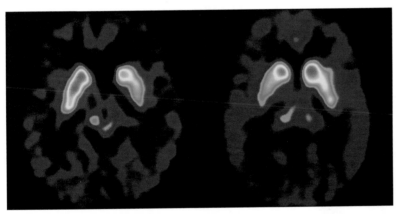

Chapter 2,
Figure 2-8, p. 22

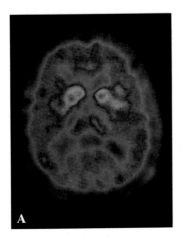
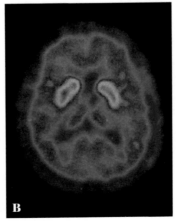
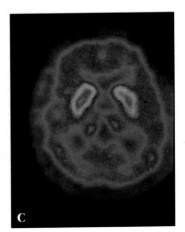

Chapter 2, Figure 2-16, p. 33

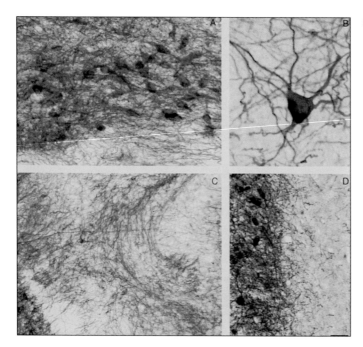

Chapter 2, Figure 2-17, p. 33

Chapter 2, Figure 2-24A, p. 38

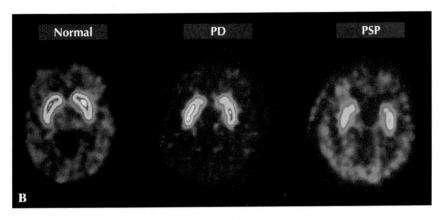

Chapter 2, Figure 2-24B, p. 38

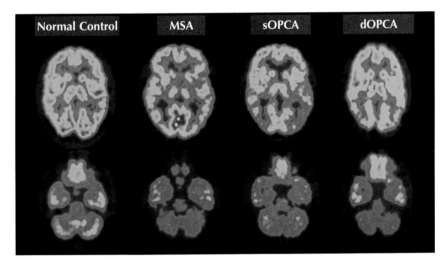

Chapter 2, Figure 2-27, p. 41

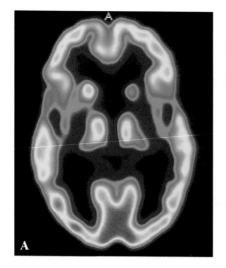 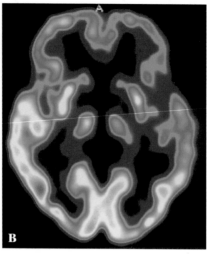

Chapter 2,
Figure 2-28, p. 42

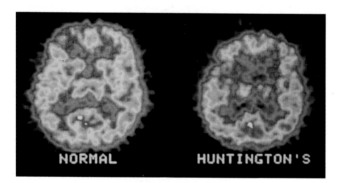

Chapter 4, Figure 4-6, p. 82

NORMAL   HUNTINGTON'S

Chapter 4, Figure 4-8C, p. 84

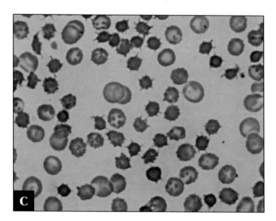